THE ULTIMATE

GOLO DIET

Cook book
for begginers

The complete guide to the Golo Diet and
healthy lifestyle

Amelia Brooks

Contents

Chapter 5. Soups 57

Chapter 6. Vegan Recipes 63

Chapter 7. Snacks Recipes **75**

Chapter 8. Dessert Recipes **80**

Exploring the Golo Diet: A Comprehensive Path to Optimal Wellness

In a world awash with diverse dietary approaches, the Golo Diet emerges as a beacon of holistic health, offering beginners a well-rounded and sustainable strategy to achieve their health and weight management goals. The Golo Diet's core premise centers around the pivotal role of stable insulin levels in optimizing metabolism. This approach harmoniously combines nutrient-dense foods, portion control, and mindful eating practices to create a holistic journey toward well-being.

Foundations of the Golo Diet

Delve deeper into the Golo Diet's foundational principles, which shape its philosophy and drive its efficacy:

Insulin Management: In stark contrast to fleeting diet trends, the Golo Diet spotlights insulin's profound impact. By meticulously selecting foods and expertly managing carbohydrate consumption, the diet seeks to stabilize insulin production. This, in turn, curtails the occurrence of energy crashes and the allure of sugar cravings, fostering a balanced internal environment.

Wholesome Nourishment: The Golo Diet champions whole foods as protagonists. With a robust lineup of lean proteins, intricate carbohydrates, healthful fats, and fiber-rich fruits and vegetables, every meal becomes an act of nourishment. This approach orchestrates a symphony of nutrients that not only satiates hunger but also cultivates holistic health and sustained vitality.

Metabolic Fuel Matrix: Pioneering the Golo Diet's culinary landscape is the innovative Metabolic Fuel Matrix. This culinary blueprint simplifies meal preparation by elucidating the perfect interplay between proteins, carbohydrates, and fats. The diet maintains a steady blood sugar trajectory by engineering this symmetrical nutrient dance, precluding unwelcome energy roller coasters.

Lifestyle Synergy: Beyond dietary choices, the Golo Diet imparts a holistic lifestyle paradigm. Regular physical activity, adept stress management, and sound sleep contribute to holistic well-being.

The Bounty of Golo Diet Benefits

In embracing the Golo Diet's tenets, novices are poised to reap a harvest of advantages:

Weight Management: The dance of insulin regulation and balanced nutrition may orchestrate a graceful weight management symphony, gently guiding individuals toward their goals.

Unwavering Energy: Steadfast blood sugar levels translate into persistent daily vitality, mitigating energy slumps and fatigue.

Blood Sugar Mastery: The Golo Diet's masterful approach to insulin management extends its embrace to blood sugar control, bestowing welcome relief for those grappling with insulin resistance.

Enhanced Metabolism: A deft interplay of Release supplements and the Metabolic Fuel Matrix sets the stage for elevated metabolic performance, bolstering fat loss endeavors.

Embarking on a Wholesome Odyssey

For those embarking on the Golo Diet odyssey, the key is a gradual transition and, if necessary, expert consultation. The Golo Diet embodies the potential for a holistic metamorphosis in eating habits, cultivating a sustainable rapport with food while placing well-being on a lofty pedestal. With the Golo Diet's intricate fusion of science, nutrition, and conscious choices, individuals unlock a gateway to a life brimming with vitality and robust health.

Elevating Wellness with Golo Diet Supplements

In the quest for holistic well-being, the Golo Diet extends its support beyond dietary choices with thoughtfully designed supplements that enhance the journey. This chapter delves into the realm of Golo Diet supplements, uncovering their role, benefits, and how they synergize with the diet's principles to amplify results and support beginners in their pursuit of optimal health.

Supplements as Catalysts for Transformation

Golo Diet supplements are not magic pills but powerful catalysts that complement the diet's philosophy and amplify its effects. These meticulously crafted formulations harness the potency of natural ingredients to address specific aspects of well-being, working in harmony with the Golo Diet's core principles.

Understanding the Golo Diet Supplement

Release: At the heart of Golo Diet supplements lies the "Release" formulation, a proprietary blend of botanical extracts and nutrients designed to enhance metabolic efficiency and manage insulin resistance. By supporting healthy insulin levels, Release assists the body in optimizing energy utilization, thereby aiding in weight management and overall health.

Enhanced Nutrient Absorption: Golo Diet supplements, including Release, are designed to optimize the absorption of essential nutrients from the foods you consume. This ensures the body efficiently utilizes nutrients for energy, immunity, and vitality.

Release: Unlocking the Potential

Insulin Management: Release is a unique blend of natural ingredients that work together to support insulin management. Enhancing insulin sensitivity and promoting balanced blood sugar levels helps prevent energy crashes, sugar cravings, and the subsequent overconsumption of calories.

Metabolic Boost: The natural ingredients in Release help boost metabolism, encouraging the body to burn stored fat for energy effectively. This synergizes with the Golo Diet's approach to creating balanced meals, supporting sustainable weight loss and enhanced vitality.

Stress Reduction: Release also includes ingredients known for their stress-reducing properties, helping to manage stress hormones that can impact weight and overall well-being.

Release Supplements: A Complementary Partner

Integration with the Golo Diet: Release supplements are designed to integrate with the Golo Diet's principles seamlessly. By incorporating Release into the dietary journey, beginners enhance the diet's effects, optimize metabolism, and experience tremendous success in weight management.

Personalized Approach: The Golo Diet recognizes that each individual's needs are unique. While Release can benefit many, consulting with healthcare professionals before starting any supplement regimen is recommended, especially for those with pre-existing health conditions or medications.

Harmonizing with Lifestyle Factors

Physical Activity: Release supplements synergize with regular physical activity, helping the body efficiently utilize energy sources during workouts and recover effectively post-exercise.

Mindful Eating: Release supplements align with the Golo Diet's emphasis on balanced and mindful eating. By supporting stable insulin levels, they maintain energy equilibrium throughout the day.

Embrace Your Enhanced Journey

Incorporating Golo Diet supplements into the wellness journey is a step towards embracing a holistic approach to well-being. By recognizing the synergy between nutrition, supplements, physical activity, and mindful choices, beginners unlock the potential for transformation beyond weight management. The Release supplement, in particular, becomes a valuable companion that supports the body's innate mechanisms, enhancing its capacity to thrive in an environment of balance, vitality, and optimal health.

Nourishing Choices: Foods to Embrace and Avoid on the Golo Diet

Embarking on the Golo Diet journey involves not just a shift in mindset but also a shift in your plate. This chapter delves into the heart of the Golo Diet, exploring the foods that align with its principles and those that are best left behind. By understanding the optimal choices for nourishment, beginners can make informed decisions that support their well-being and lay the foundation for a healthier life.

A Symphony of Nutrient-Rich Foods

Lean Proteins: Embrace lean protein sources, such as skinless poultry, lean cuts of meat and seafood, and plant-based options like tofu and legumes. These proteins provide vital amino acids that support muscle growth, repair, and overall vitality. Poultry are excellent choices as they are lower in saturated fat than red meats.

Complex Carbohydrates: Opt for complex carbohydrates with a lower glycemic index, including whole grains like quinoa, brown rice, and whole wheat. These carbohydrates release energy gradually, promoting stable blood sugar levels and sustained energy throughout the day. Whole grains are rich in fiber, which helps you feel full longer.

Fiber-Rich Fruits and Vegetables: Load your plate with colorful fruits and vegetables. These vibrant foods are rich in fiber, vitamins, minerals, and antioxidants that support digestion, immunity, and overall health. Berries, leafy greens, and cruciferous vegetables like broccoli and cauliflower are especially beneficial.

Healthy Fats: Incorporate sources of healthy fats such as avocados, nuts, seeds, and olive oil. These fats provide satiety, aid nutrient absorption, and support heart health. Omega-3 fatty acids in fish like salmon and chia seeds offer anti-inflammatory benefits.

Navigating the Golo Diet: What to Include

The Metabolic Fuel Matrix: Craft your meals using the Metabolic Fuel Matrix, balancing proteins, carbohydrates, and fats in the appropriate ratios. This framework ensures that your body receives a harmonious blend of nutrients that optimize energy and support metabolism. For example, a breakfast of scrambled eggs with spinach and avocado on whole-grain toast is a balanced option.

Portion Control: Embrace portion control as a cornerstone of the Golo Diet. Pay attention to serving sizes to prevent overeating and ensure you're consuming an appropriate amount of calories for your needs. Use small plates to help manage portion sizes.

Release Supplements: Consider incorporating Release supplements into your routine to enhance insulin management and metabolic efficiency. These supplements complement the Golo Diet's principles, helping you achieve your wellness goals more effectively. Consult a healthcare professional before adding suplements to your diet.

Steering Clear: Foods to Avoid

Refined Sugars: Minimize or eliminate foods high in refined sugars, such as sugary beverages, candies, and baked goods. These foods can lead to rapid spikes and crashes in blood sugar levels, hindering your efforts to stabilize energy and manage weight. Opt for whole fruit for natural sweetness.

Processed Foods: Reduce your intake of processed and highly processed foods, which often contain hidden sugars, unhealthy fats, and artificial additives that don't align with the Golo Diet's focus on wholesome nutrition. Read ingredient labels and choose foods with minimal additives.

Excessive Sodium: Be mindful of sodium intake by avoiding heavily salted foods. High sodium consumption can contribute to bloating and elevated blood pressure. Opt for fresh or minimally processed foods and use herbs and spices for flavor.

Embrace the Golo Diet Lifestyle

The Golo Diet isn't just about what you eat—it's a lifestyle that encourages you to prioritize your health and well-being. By nourishing your body with nutrient-rich foods, balancing macronutrients, and adopting mindful eating habits, you're setting yourself up for success on your journey toward vitality and optimal health. Everyone's dietary needs are unique, so listening to your body and consulting a healthcare professional is essential.

Benefits of the Golo Diet

As you embark on your journey with the Golo Diet, you're not just embracing a new way of eating—you're opening the door to a world of health and well-being. This chapter dives into the numerous benefits of the Golo Diet, showcasing how its principles can positively impact your body, mind, and overall quality of life.

Steady Energy Throughout the Day

One of the Golo Diet's most noticeable benefits is its consistent energy. By focusing on stable blood sugar levels through controlled carbohydrate intake and nutrient-rich foods, you can bid farewell to energy crashes and the infamous midday slumps. Say hello to sustained vitality that supports your productivity and keeps you alert and focused throughout the day.

Healthy Weight Management

The Golo Diet's approach to insulin regulation plays a pivotal role in supporting healthy weight management. By managing blood sugar levels, you can effectively reduce cravings for sugary and processed foods, leading to more controlled eating habits. With an emphasis on portion control and balanced nutrition, the Golo Diet can help you achieve and maintain a healthy weight over time.

Improved Blood Sugar Control

For individuals with insulin resistance or pre-diabetes, the Golo Diet can be particularly beneficial. By choosing foods that support stable blood sugar levels, you can better manage your glucose metabolism and reduce the risk of blood sugar spikes and crashes. This can improve insulin sensitivity, ultimately supporting better overall blood sugar control.

Enhanced Metabolism and Fat Loss

The Golo Diet's approach to combining proteins, carbohydrates, and fats in the Metabolic Fuel Matrix can help enhance your metabolism. This means your body becomes more efficient at burning calories, aiding fat loss, and promoting lean muscle mass. Incorporating Release supplements can further support your metabolism, contributing to your weight management goals.

Heart Health and Inflammation Reduction

The Golo Diet aligns with heart-healthy dietary patterns, focusing on incorporating healthy fats, lean proteins, and whole grains. By choosing foods rich in omega-3 fatty acids, antioxidants, and fiber, you can help reduce inflammation and support cardiovascular health. Lowering inflammation also has broader health implications, potentially reducing the risk of chronic diseases.

Better Digestion and Gut Health

The fiber-rich fruits, vegetables, and whole grains encouraged by the Golo Diet promote optimal digestion and gut health. Fiber supports regular bowel movements, prevents constipation, and contributes to a healthy gut microbiome. A balanced gut microbiome is linked to improved digestion, nutrient absorption, and mental well-being.

Mindful Eating and Improved Relationship with Food

The Golo Diet's emphasis on mindful eating encourages you to savor each bite, listen to your body's hunger and fullness cues, and foster a healthier relationship with food. By cultivating mindfulness around eating, you can break free from emotional eating habits, better understand your body's needs, and make choices that align with your goals.

Boosted Immunity and Nutrient Intake

The Golo Diet's focus on nutrient-dense foods means you provide your body with the vitamins, minerals, and antioxidants needed to maintain a strong immune system. A diet rich in fruits and vegetables can help protect your body against illness and enhance your overall well-being.

A Holistic Approach to Wellness

The benefits of the Golo Diet extend beyond physical health. By embracing a balanced lifestyle that includes regular physical activity, stress management, and ample sleep, you're cultivating a holistic approach to well-being. The Golo Diet is a foundation for making mindful choices that support your overall quality of life.

Your Journey to Well-Being

Remember that the benefits of the Golo Diet are not one-size-fits-all. Each individual's experience may vary based on metabolism, health conditions, and lifestyle. It's important to listen to your body, be patient with your progress, and seek guidance from healthcare professionals as needed. As you continue your Golo Diet journey, celebrate the positive changes you experience and the newfound sense of empowerment that comes with making nourishing choices.

Exploring Possible Limitations of the Golo Diet

While the Golo Diet offers a holistic and balanced approach to wellness, it's essential to consider that no diet is without its potential drawbacks. In this chapter, we'll delve into some potential downsides of the Golo Diet, ensuring you have a comprehensive understanding before embarking on your dietary journey.

Initial Adjustment Period

Transitioning to the Golo Diet may involve adjusting as your body adapts to new eating patterns. You might experience changes in digestion, energy levels, and cravings. During this phase, it's essential to be patient with yourself and allow your body to acclimate to the changes.

Restriction of Certain Foods

While the Golo Diet promotes nutrient-rich whole foods, it does limit or discourage the consumption of certain foods. This could lead to feelings of deprivation or difficulty in social situations where these foods are prevalent. It's vital to balance adhering to the diet's principles and enjoying occasional treats.

Individual Variability

Our bodies respond differently to dietary changes due to genetics, metabolism, and health conditions. While some individuals may experience significant benefits from the Golo Diet, others might not achieve the same results. Managing expectations and prioritizing overall well-being over solely focusing on weight loss is essential.

Nutrient Considerations

The Golo Diet encourages a variety of nutrient-dense foods, but there's potential for nutrient imbalances if not carefully planned. For instance, supplementation might be necessary if you must be more intentional about obtaining specific vitamins or minerals, such as vitamin B12 or iron. Consulting a healthcare professional can help you make informed choices about supplementation.

Social Challenges

Following the Golo Diet might present challenges in social settings or dining out. It's common to feel isolated or self-conscious when your dietary choices differ from those around you. Additionally, the transition might require extra effort and time if you need to familiarize yourself with meal planning or cooking from scratch.

Monitoring Health

If you have underlying health conditions, monitoring your health closely while on the Golo Diet is crucial. While the diet aims to stabilize blood sugar levels, individuals with diabetes or other medical conditions must work closely with healthcare providers to manage medication dosages and ensure optimal health.

Flexibility and Long-Term Sustainability

Due to its restrictions and guidelines, the Golo Diet's specific approach might be challenging to sustain over the long term. While it can provide short-term benefits, some individuals might need help to incorporate it into their lifestyles indefinitely. Exploring ways to maintain a balanced and varied diet while adhering to the diet's core principles is essential for lasting success.

Enhancing Your Diet Journey: Tips for Optimal Results

Embarking on a diet journey, such as the Golo Diet, is a commitment to your health and well-being. While the diet itself provides a solid foundation, there are several strategies you can implement to maximize your results and ensure a successful experience. In this chapter, we'll explore actionable steps you can take to enhance your diet journey and achieve your goals.

1. Stay Hydrated

Water plays a crucial role in supporting metabolism and maintaining overall health. Ensure you're drinking an adequate amount of water throughout the day to stay hydrated. Herbal teas, infused water, and electrolyte-rich beverages can also contribute to your hydration efforts.

2. Prioritize sleep

Quality sleep is essential for weight management and overall well-being. Aim for 7-9 hours of restful sleep each night. Establish a relaxing bedtime routine, create a comfortable sleep environment, and limit screen time before bed to promote better sleep quality.

3. Move Regularly

Physical activity complements your dietary efforts by boosting metabolism, enhancing mood, and supporting weight loss. Incorporate both cardiovascular exercises and strength training into your routine. Find activities you enjoy and aim for at least 150 minutes of moderate-intensity exercise each week.

4. Mindful Eating

Practicing mindful eating encourages you to savor each bite and tune into your body's hunger and fullness cues. Avoid distractions while eating, chew your food thoroughly, and take time to appreciate the flavors and textures of your meals.

5. Manage stress

Chronic stress can hinder weight loss and overall well-being. Engage in stress-reduction techniques such as meditation, deep breathing, yoga, or spending time in nature. Finding healthy outlets for stress can positively impact your results.

6. Plan and Prep

Meal planning and preparation set the stage for dietary success. Plan your meals and snacks ahead of time, batch cook, and have nutritious options readily available to avoid making impulsive choices when hunger strikes.

7. Listen to Your Body

Pay attention to how different foods make you feel. Notice if certain foods cause discomfort, bloating, or energy crashes. Adjust your food choices based on your body's signals to optimize your dietary experience.

8. Stay Consistent

Consistency is critical to achieving your goals. Stick to the Golo Diet's principles and avoid extreme restriction or binge-eating episodes. Gradual and sustainable changes yield long-lasting results.

9. Seek support

Enlist the support of friends, family, or online communities that share your dietary goals. Sharing your journey and exchanging tips and experiences can provide motivation and accountability.

10. Track progress

Document your progress to stay motivated and track your achievements. Keep a journal, take measurements, or snap photos to observe your changes visually. Celebrate your milestones along the way.

Essential Kitchen Tools for Your Golo Diet Journey

Equipping your kitchen with the right tools can make your Golo Diet journey smoother, more efficient, and enjoyable. Whether you're a seasoned chef or a beginner, having the following recommended kitchen tools will help you prepare nutritious and delicious meals that align with the Golo Diet's principles.

1. Food Scale

A food scale is invaluable for accurately measuring portion sizes and ingredients. It helps you maintain portion control and ensures you follow the Golo Diet's guidelines for balanced meals.

2. Measuring Cups and Spoons

Precise measurements are crucial for creating recipes that align with the Golo Diet's principles. Measuring cups and spoons enable you to portion ingredients accurately, especially when cooking or baking.

3. Blender or Food Processor

Blenders and food processors are versatile tools that can help you create smoothies, sauces, dressings, and nut butter using whole ingredients. They make it easy to incorporate nutrient-rich foods into your diet.

4. Steamer Basket

Steaming is a healthy cooking method that preserves the nutrients in vegetables and proteins. A steamer basket allows you to cook vegetables, fish, and poultry without adding fats.

5. Non-Stick Cookware

Non-stick pans and pots are essential for cooking with minimal oil or fat. They prevent sticking and make it easier to sauté, stir-fry, and cook proteins without excessive grease.

6. Baking Sheet and Parchment Paper

Baking sheets and parchment paper are helpful for roasting vegetables, baking proteins, and preparing healthy snacks. They make cleanup a breeze and ensure even cooking.

7. Spiralizer

A spiralizer is a fun and innovative tool that turns vegetables like zucchini, carrots, and sweet potatoes into noodle-like strands. It's perfect for creating low-carb pasta alternatives.

8. Salad Spinner

A salad spinner makes washing and drying leafy greens quick and efficient. It helps you prepare fresh and crisp salads without excess moisture.

9. Herb Scissors or Chopper

Fresh herbs add flavor and nutrients to your meals. Herb scissors or a chopper make it easy to chop herbs, finely enhancing your dishes' taste.

10. Cutting Board Set

A set of cutting boards in different sizes and materials (wood, plastic, or bamboo) helps you keep your food prep organized and prevents cross-contamination.

11. Kitchen Thermometer

A kitchen thermometer ensures that proteins are cooked to the proper internal temperature, reducing the risk of undercooked meat and ensuring food safety.

12. Citrus Juicer or Reamer

Fresh citrus juice adds zing to dressings, marinades, and beverages. A citrus juicer or reamer extracts juice efficiently without seeds.

13. Mixing Bowls

A variety of mixing bowls in different sizes is essential for meal prep, tossing salads, and mixing ingredients for recipes.

14. Grater or Microplane

Graters and microplates are handy for adding grated cheese, zest, or finely grated vegetables to your dishes.

15. High-Quality Chef's Knife

Invest in a sharp and versatile chef's knife for slicing, dicing, and chopping. A good knife makes food prep safer and more efficient.

16. Storage Containers

High-quality storage containers help you store leftovers, prepped ingredients, and snacks while keeping them fresh and organized.

17. Slow Cooker or Instant Pot

A slow cooker or Instant Pot can save time and energy while preparing soups, stews, and one-pot meals that align with the Golo Diet's principles.

18. Whisk and mix utensils

Whisks and mixing utensils are essential for blending ingredients, whisking dressings, and mixing in your recipes.

Building a Well-Equipped Kitchen

The right kitchen tools can empower you to create wholesome and satisfying meals supporting your Golo Diet journey. As you gather these essential items, remember that a well-equipped kitchen enhances your cooking experience and encourages you to explore new recipes and enjoy nourishing yourself and your loved ones.

Almond Butter Banana Pancakes

Serving: 4 | Prep time: 10 minutes | Cook time: 15 minutes

Ingredients:

- 7 oz (200 g) ripe bananas, mashed
- 3 large eggs
- 2 oz (60 g) almond butter
- 1 tsp vanilla extract
- 2 oz (60 g) almond flour
- 0.5 tsp baking powder
- 0.25 tsp cinnamon
- Pinch of salt
- Coconut oil for cooking

Directions:

1. In a mixing bowl, combine the mashed bananas, eggs, almond butter, and vanilla extract until well blended.
2. Add the almond flour, baking powder, cinnamon, and salt to the bowl; mix until a smooth batter forms.
3. Heat a non-stick skillet over medium-low heat and lightly grease it with coconut oil.
4. Pour approximately 1/4 cup of batter onto the skillet for each pancake. Cook until bubbles form on the surface, then flip and cook the other side until golden brown.
5. Repeat until all the batter is used.
6. Serve the pancakes warm, topped with fresh banana slices, a drizzle of almond butter, and a sprinkle of cinnamon.

Nutritional Values: Calories: 265 kcal | Fat: 17 g | Protein: 10 g | Carbs: 19 g | Net carbs: 10 g | Fiber: 9 g | Cholesterol: 186 mg | Sodium: 127 mg | Potassium: 329 mg

Useful Tip: To add a nutritional boost, consider sprinkling some chia seeds or ground flaxseeds onto the batter before cooking for extra fiber and omega-3 fatty acids.

Chia Berry Breakfast Parfait

Serving: 4 | Prep time: 10 minutes | Cook time: 0 minutes

Ingredients:

- 2 oz (57 g) chia seeds
- 16 oz (473 ml) unsweetened almond milk
- 1 tsp vanilla extract
- 6 oz (170 g) mixed berries (strawberries, blueberries, raspberries)
- 8 oz (227 g) Greek yogurt (unsweetened)
- 1 oz (28 g) chopped nuts (almonds, walnuts, or your choice)
- 0.5 oz (14 g) unsweetened shredded coconut

Directions:

1. In a mixing bowl, combine chia seeds, almond milk, and vanilla extract, stirring well to prevent clumps; let it sit for about 15 minutes until it thickens into a pudding-like consistency.
2. Create a berry compote by mashing half of the mixed berries in a bowl.
3. Layer the ingredients in serving glasses or bowls: Begin with a layer of chia seed pudding, followed by a layer of berry compote, a spoonful of Greek yogurt, and a sprinkle of chopped nuts.
4. Repeat the layers until your glasses are full, ending with a dollop of Greek yogurt on top and a sprinkle of shredded coconut.
5. Refrigerate the parfaits for at least 30 minutes before serving, allowing the flavors to meld.

Nutritional Values: Calories: 248 kcal | Fat: 11 g | Protein: 10 g | Carbs: 28 g | Net carbs: 14 g | Fiber: 14 g | Cholesterol: 3 mg | Sodium: 67 mg | Potassium: 378 mg

Useful Tip: For an added crunch and nutritional boost, consider adding a tablespoon of ground flaxseeds or pumpkin seeds between the layers.

Sweet Potato Hash with Turkey Sausage

Serving: 4 | Prep time: 15 minutes | Cook time: 25 minutes

Ingredients:

- 16 oz (454 g) sweet potatoes, peeled and diced
- 10 oz (283 g) lean turkey sausage, casings removed
- 1 medium onion, chopped
- 1 red bell pepper, diced
- 2 cloves garlic, minced
- 2 tbsp olive oil
- 1 tsp smoked paprika
- 0.5 tsp ground cumin
- Salt and pepper to taste
- Fresh parsley, chopped (for garnish)

Directions:

1. Heat 1 tablespoon of olive oil in a large skillet over medium heat.
2. Add the turkey sausage and cook, breaking it into crumbles, until browned and cooked through. Remove the sausage from the skillet and set aside.
3. In the same skillet, add the remaining tablespoon of olive oil. Add the diced sweet potatoes and cook for about 10 minutes, or until they start to soften and develop a golden crust.
4. Add the chopped onion and red bell pepper to the skillet. Sauté for another 5 minutes until the vegetables are tender.
5. Stir in the minced garlic, smoked paprika, and ground cumin, and cook for an additional 1-2 minutes until fragrant.
6. Return the cooked turkey sausage to the skillet and mix well with the sweet potato mixture. Cook for another 3-4 minutes to allow the flavors to meld.
7. Season the hash with salt and pepper to taste.
8. Garnish with chopped fresh parsley before serving.

Nutritional Values: Calories: 312 kcal | Fat: 15 g | Protein: 20 g | Carbs: 26 g | Net carbs: 20 g | Fiber: 6 g | Cholesterol: 52 mg | Sodium: 712 mg | Potassium: 700 mg

Useful Tip: For an extra boost of flavor, you can top the sweet potato hash with a dollop of Greek yogurt and a sprinkle of hot sauce.

Cinnamon Raisin Oatmeal with Pecans

Serving: 4 | Prep time: 5 minutes | Cook time: 15 minutes

Ingredients:

- 4 oz (113 g) old-fashioned rolled oats
- 16 oz (473 ml) water
- 8 oz (237 ml) unsweetened almond milk
- 1 tsp ground cinnamon
- 2.5 oz (71 g) raisins
- 1 oz (28 g) chopped pecans
- 1 tbsp maple syrup (optional)
- Pinch of salt

Directions:

1. In a medium-sized pot, combine the rolled oats, water, and almond milk.
2. Bring the mixture to a boil over medium-high heat, then reduce the heat to low and simmer for about 10-12 minutes, stirring occasionally, until the oats are tender and the mixture thickens.
3. Stir in the ground cinnamon and a pinch of salt.
4. Remove the pot from the heat and stir in the raisins and chopped pecans.
5. If desired, drizzle with maple syrup for added sweetness.
6. Divide the oatmeal into serving bowls and enjoy warm.

Nutritional Values: Calories: 248 kcal | Fat: 8 g | Protein: 6 g | Carbs: 40 g | Net carbs: 31 g | Fiber: 9 g | Cholesterol: 0 mg | Sodium: 92 mg | Potassium: 248 mg

Useful Tip: To add extra flavor and nutrients, consider stirring in a tablespoon of ground flaxseeds or chia seeds after cooking.

Spinach and Feta Egg White Scramble

Serving: 4 | Prep time: 10 minutes | Cook time: 10 minutes

Ingredients:

- 8 oz (227 g) fresh spinach, washed and chopped
- 16 oz (473 ml) egg whites
- 4 oz (113 g) crumbled feta cheese
- 1 medium tomato, diced
- 1/2 medium red onion, finely chopped
- 2 cloves garlic, minced
- 1 tbsp olive oil
- 1/2 tsp dried oregano
- Salt and pepper to taste
- Fresh parsley, chopped (for garnish)

Directions:

1. In a large skillet, heat the olive oil over medium heat.
2. Add the chopped red onion and sauté for about 2-3 minutes until softened.
3. Stir in the minced garlic and cook for an additional 30 seconds until fragrant.
4. Add the diced tomato to the skillet and cook for 2 minutes until slightly softened.
5. Add the chopped spinach to the skillet and cook for another 2-3 minutes until wilted.
6. Pour in the egg whites and scramble them with the vegetables, cooking until they are fully set.
7. Stir in the crumbled feta cheese and dried oregano; season with salt and pepper to taste.
8. Once the cheese is slightly melted, remove the skillet from heat.
9. Garnish the scramble with chopped fresh parsley before serving.

Nutritional Values: Calories: 167 kcal | Fat: 8 g | Protein: 16 g | Carbs: 8 g | Net carbs: 5 g | Fiber: 3 g | Cholesterol: 20 mg | Sodium: 494 mg | Potassium: 494 mg

Useful Tip: For an extra protein boost, consider adding some diced cooked chicken or turkey breast to the scramble.

Blueberry Coconut Flour Waffles

Serving: 4 | Prep time: 10 minutes | Cook time: 15 minutes

Ingredients:

- 3 oz (85 g) coconut flour
- 1 tsp baking powder
- 1/4 tsp salt
- 4 large eggs
- 4 oz (120 ml) unsweetened almond milk
- 2 tbsp coconut oil, melted
- 1 tbsp maple syrup (optional)
- 2.5 oz (71 g) blueberries
- Coconut oil or cooking spray for waffle iron

Directions:

1. Preheat your waffle iron according to the manufacturer's instructions.
2. In a bowl, whisk together the coconut flour, baking powder, and salt.
3. In another bowl, beat the eggs, then add almond milk, melted coconut oil, and maple syrup (if using), and mix well.
4. Combine the wet and dry ingredients, stirring until a smooth batter forms.
5. Gently fold in the blueberries.
6. Lightly grease the waffle iron with coconut oil or cooking spray.
7. Pour an appropriate amount of batter onto the preheated waffle iron and cook until golden brown and crisp.
8. Repeat with the remaining batter.
9. Serve the waffles warm, topped with additional blueberries and a drizzle of maple syrup if desired.

Nutritional Values: Calories: 197 kcal | Fat: 11 g | Protein: 7 g | Carbs: 18 g | Net carbs: 6 g | Fiber: 12 g | Cholesterol: 186 mg | Sodium: 281 mg | Potassium: 272 mg

Useful Tip: To enhance the waffle's nutritional profile, you can add a tablespoon of ground flaxseeds or chia seeds to the batter.

Zucchini and Mushroom Breakfast Quesadilla

Serving: 4 | Prep time: 15 minutes | Cook time: 15 minutes

Ingredients:

- 4 medium zucchinis, grated
- 8 oz (227 g) mushrooms, sliced
- 1 medium red onion, thinly sliced
- 2 cloves garlic, minced
- 4 whole-wheat tortillas
- 4 oz (113 g) low-fat mozzarella cheese, shredded
- 2 tbsp olive oil
- 1 tsp dried thyme
- Salt and pepper to taste
- Cooking spray

Directions:

1. Heat 1 tablespoon of olive oil in a large skillet over medium heat.
2. Add the sliced mushrooms and cook until they release their moisture and turn golden brown, about 5-7 minutes. Remove from the skillet and set aside.
3. In the same skillet, add the remaining tablespoon of olive oil. Sauté the sliced red onion until softened, about 2-3 minutes.
4. Add the minced garlic and cook for an additional 30 seconds until fragrant.
5. Add the grated zucchini to the skillet and cook for about 5-6 minutes, stirring occasionally, until most of the moisture has evaporated.
6. Stir in the cooked mushrooms, dried thyme, salt, and pepper. Mix well and remove from heat.
7. Preheat another skillet over medium heat and lightly grease it with cooking spray.
8. Place a tortilla in the skillet and sprinkle half of the shredded mozzarella cheese over one half of the tortilla.
9. Spoon a portion of the zucchini and mushroom mixture onto the cheese, then fold the tortilla in half.
10. Cook the quesadilla for about 2-3 minutes on each side, until the tortilla is crispy and the cheese is melted.
11. Repeat the process for the remaining tortillas and filling.
12. Slice the quesadillas into wedges and serve warm.

Nutritional Values: Calories: 257 kcal | Fat: 9 g | Protein: 12 g | Carbs: 36 g | Net carbs: 30 g | Fiber: 6 g | Cholesterol: 15 mg | Sodium: 371 mg | Potassium: 841 mg

Useful Tip: To add a touch of freshness, serve the quesadillas with a side of salsa or sliced avocado.

Apple Cinnamon Breakfast Quinoa

Serving: 4 | Prep time: 10 minutes | Cook time: 20 minutes

Ingredients:

- 8 oz (227 g) quinoa, rinsed and drained
- 16 oz (473 ml) unsweetened almond milk
- 2 medium apples, peeled, cored, and diced
- 1 tsp ground cinnamon
- 1/4 tsp nutmeg
- 1 oz (28 g) chopped walnuts
- 2 tbsp maple syrup (optional)
- Pinch of salt

Directions:

1. In a medium pot, combine the quinoa and almond milk.
2. Bring the mixture to a boil over medium-high heat, then reduce the heat to low, cover, and simmer for about 15 minutes, or until the quinoa is cooked and the liquid is absorbed.
3. While the quinoa is cooking, heat a non-stick skillet over medium heat.
4. Add the diced apples, ground cinnamon, and nutmeg to the skillet. Cook for about 5-7 minutes until the apples are tender and slightly caramelized.
5. Once the quinoa is cooked, fluff it with a fork and stir in the cooked apples and chopped walnuts.
6. If desired, drizzle with maple syrup for added sweetness.
7. Season with a pinch of salt and additional cinnamon if preferred.
8. Serve the breakfast quinoa warm.

Nutritional Values: Calories: 290 kcal | Fat: 10 g | Protein: 8 g | Carbs: 43 g | Net carbs: 34 g | Fiber: 9 g | Cholesterol: 0 mg | Sodium: 159 mg | Potassium: 410 mg

Useful Tip: Customize your breakfast quinoa by adding a dollop of Greek yogurt and a sprinkle of chia seeds or flaxseeds for extra protein and omega-3 fatty acids.

Mediterranean-style Veggie Omelette

Serving: 4 | Prep time: 10 minutes | Cook time: 15 minutes

Ingredients:

- 8 large eggs
- 4 oz (113 g) baby spinach
- 1 medium red bell pepper, diced
- 1 small zucchini , diced
- 2 oz (57 g) crumbled feta cheese
- 1 oz (28 g) sliced black olives
- 2 tbsp olive oil
- 1 tsp dried oregano
- Salt and pepper to taste

Directions:

1. In a bowl, whisk the eggs until well combined, and season with a pinch of salt and pepper.
2. Heat 1 tablespoon of olive oil in a non-stick skillet over medium heat.
3. Add the diced red bell pepper and zucchini to the skillet and sauté for about 5 minutes until softened.
4. Add the baby spinach to the skillet and cook for an additional 2-3 minutes until wilted.
5. Remove the vegetables from the skillet and set aside.
6. Wipe the skillet clean, add the remaining tablespoon of olive oil, and heat it over medium heat.
7. Pour half of the beaten eggs into the skillet, swirling to evenly distribute.
8. Once the edges of the omelette are set, spread half of the cooked vegetables, feta cheese, and sliced olives on one half of the omelette.
9. Sprinkle with dried oregano and fold the other half of the omelette over the filling.
10. Cook for another 2-3 minutes until the omelette is fully cooked and the cheese is slightly melted.
11. Slide the omelette onto a plate and repeat the process to make a second omelette.
12. Garnish with additional feta cheese and olives if desired.

Nutritional Values: Calories: 245 kcal | Fat: 18 g | Protein: 14 g | Carbs: 8 g | Net carbs: 5 g | Fiber: 3 g | Cholesterol: 372 mg | Sodium: 620 mg | Potassium: 463 mg

Useful Tip: Serve the omelettes with a side of whole-grain toast or a mixed greens salad for a well-rounded breakfast.

Bacon and Spinach Stuffed Portobello Mushrooms

Serving: 4 | Prep time: 15 minutes | Cook time: 20 minutes

Ingredients:

- 4 large Portobello mushrooms
- 4 slices of turkey bacon, cooked and crumbled
- 4 oz (113 g) baby spinach
- 2 oz (57 g) shredded mozzarella cheese
- 1 oz (28 g) grated Parmesan cheese
- 2 cloves garlic, minced
- 2 tbsp olive oil
- Salt and pepper to taste
- Fresh parsley, chopped (for garnish)

Directions:

1. Preheat the oven to 375°F (190°C).
2. Remove the stems from the Portobello mushrooms and gently scrape out the gills using a spoon. Place the mushrooms on a baking sheet.
3. In a skillet, heat the olive oil over medium heat. Add the minced garlic and sauté for about 1 minute until fragrant.
4. Add the baby spinach to the skillet and cook until wilted, about 2-3 minutes. Remove from heat.
5. In a bowl, combine the cooked and crumbled turkey bacon, wilted spinach, shredded mozzarella cheese, grated Parmesan cheese, salt, and pepper.
6. Divide the bacon and spinach mixture evenly among the Portobello mushrooms, filling each cap.
7. Place the stuffed mushrooms in the preheated oven and bake for about 15-20 minutes, or until the mushrooms are tender and the cheese is melted and bubbly.
8. Remove from the oven and garnish with chopped fresh parsley before serving.

Nutritional Values: Calories: 182 kcal | Fat: 11 g | Protein: 16 g | Carbs: 8 g | Net carbs: 4 g | Fiber: 4 g | Cholesterol: 28 mg | Sodium: 414 mg | Potassium: 915 mg

Useful Tip: To add an extra layer of flavor, sprinkle a pinch of red pepper flakes over the stuffed mushrooms before baking.

Flaxseed Banana Muffins with Walnuts

Serving: 4 | Prep time: 15 minutes | Cook time: 25 minutes

Ingredients:

- 6 oz (170 g) ripe bananas (about 2 medium bananas), mashed
- 2 oz (56 g) ground flaxseed
- 2 oz (56 g) almond flour
- 2 large eggs
- 2 oz (57 g) unsweetened applesauce
- 2 oz (60 ml) unsweetened almond milk
- 1 oz (28 g) chopped walnuts
- 2 tbsp maple syrup (optional)
- 1 tsp baking powder
- 1 tsp ground cinnamon
- 1/2 tsp vanilla extract
- Pinch of salt

Directions:

1. Preheat the oven to 350°F (175°C) and line a muffin tin with paper liners.
2. In a bowl, whisk together the mashed bananas, eggs, unsweetened applesauce, almond milk, maple syrup (if using), and vanilla extract.
3. In another bowl, combine the ground flaxseed, almond flour, baking powder, ground cinnamon, and a pinch of salt.
4. Mix the wet ingredients into the dry ingredients until just combined.
5. Gently fold in the chopped walnuts.
6. Divide the batter evenly among the muffin cups, filling each about 3/4 full.
7. Bake in the preheated oven for 20-25 minutes, or until a toothpick inserted into the center of a muffin comes out clean.
8. Allow the muffins to cool in the tin for a few minutes before transferring them to a wire rack to cool completely.

Nutritional Values: Calories: 231 kcal | Fat: 17 g | Protein: 7 g | Carbs: 15 g | Net carbs: 5 g | Fiber: 10 g | Cholesterol: 81 mg | Sodium: 80 mg | Potassium: 347 mg

Useful Tip: For added crunch and nutrition, sprinkle a few extra chopped walnuts on top of each muffin before baking.

Smoked Salmon and Cream Cheese Stuffed Bell Peppers

Serving: 4 | Prep time: 15 minutes | Cook time: 20 minutes

Ingredients:

- 4 large bell peppers (assorted colors)
- 4 oz (113 g) smoked salmon, thinly sliced
- 4 oz (113 g) low-fat cream cheese, softened
- 1 oz (28 g) red onion, finely chopped
- 2 tbsp fresh lemon juice
- 1 tbsp capers, drained and chopped
- 1 tbsp fresh dill, chopped
- Salt and pepper to taste

Directions:

1. Preheat the oven to 375°F (190°C).
2. Slice the tops off the bell peppers and remove the seeds and membranes. Rinse and pat dry.
3. In a bowl, combine the softened cream cheese, chopped red onion, fresh lemon juice, chopped capers, and fresh dill. Mix well.
4. Gently fold in the smoked salmon into the cream cheese mixture.
5. Season the mixture with salt and pepper to taste.
6. Stuff the bell peppers with the cream cheese and smoked salmon mixture, pressing down gently to fill.
7. Place the stuffed peppers on a baking dish and bake in the preheated oven for 20-25 minutes, or until the peppers are tender and the filling is heated through.
8. Remove from the oven and let cool slightly before serving.

Nutritional Values: Calories: 186 kcal | Fat: 10 g | Protein: 13 g | Carbs: 11 g | Net carbs: 8 g | Fiber: 3 g | Cholesterol: 36 mg | Sodium: 579 mg | Potassium: 489 mg

Useful Tip: Serve these stuffed peppers with a side salad or a slice of whole-grain bread for a complete and satisfying breakfast.

Turmeric Infused Golden Omelette

Serving: 4 | Prep time: 10 minutes | Cook time: 10 minutes

Ingredients:

- 8 large eggs
- 1/2 tsp ground turmeric
- 1/4 tsp ground cumin
- 1 oz (28 g) grated cheddar cheese
- 1 oz (28 g) diced red bell pepper
- 1 oz (28 g) diced onion
- 2 tbsp unsweetened almond milk
- 1 tbsp olive oil
- Salt and pepper to taste
- Fresh cilantro, chopped (for garnish)

Directions:

1. In a bowl, whisk together the eggs, ground turmeric, ground cumin, unsweetened almond milk, and a pinch of salt and pepper.
2. Heat the olive oil in a non-stick skillet over medium heat.
3. Add the diced red bell pepper and onion to the skillet and sauté for about 3-4 minutes until softened.
4. Pour the egg mixture into the skillet, swirling to evenly distribute.
5. Sprinkle the grated cheddar cheese over one half of the omelette.
6. Cook the omelette for 2-3 minutes until the edges are set and the cheese is slightly melted.
7. Fold the other half of the omelette over the cheese-filled side.
8. Cook for another 2-3 minutes until the omelette is fully cooked.
9. Slide the omelette onto a plate, garnish with chopped cilantro, and serve.

Nutritional Values: Calories: 195 kcal | Fat: 13 g | Protein: 15 g | Carbs: 3 g | Net carbs: 2 g | Fiber: 1 g | Cholesterol: 374 mg | Sodium: 252 mg | Potassium: 214 mg

Useful Tip: Turmeric is known for its anti-inflammatory properties; feel free to add a pinch of black pepper to enhance its absorption.

Quinoa and Black Bean Breakfast Burrito

Serving: 4 | Prep time: 15 minutes | Cook time: 20 minutes

Ingredients:

- 4 large whole-grain tortillas
- 6.5 oz (185 g) cooked quinoa
- 6 oz (165 g) cooked black beans, drained and rinsed
- 2 oz (57 g) diced red bell pepper
- 1 oz (28 g) diced red onion
- 2 oz (57 g) diced tomatoes
- 2 oz (57 g) shredded cheddar cheese
- 4 large eggs, scrambled
- 2 tbsp olive oil
- 1 tsp ground cumin
- 1/2 tsp chili powder
- Salt and pepper to taste
- Fresh cilantro, chopped (for garnish)
- Salsa or hot sauce (optional, for serving)

Directions:

1. In a skillet, heat the olive oil over medium heat.
2. Add the diced red bell pepper and red onion to the skillet and sauté for about 3-4 minutes until softened.
3. Stir in the cooked black beans, ground cumin, chili powder, salt, and pepper. Cook for another 2 minutes to heat the beans.
4. In a separate pan, scramble the eggs until cooked to your preference.
5. Warm the tortillas in a dry skillet or microwave.
6. To assemble, place a tortilla on a flat surface. Layer with cooked quinoa, black bean mixture, scrambled eggs, diced tomatoes, shredded cheddar cheese, and chopped cilantro.
7. Fold in the sides of the tortilla and then roll it up tightly to create a burrito.
8. Repeat with the remaining tortillas and ingredients.
9. Serve the burritos with salsa or hot sauce on the side, if desired.

Nutritional Values: Calories: 358 kcal | Fat: 17 g | Protein: 17 g | Carbs: 37 g | Net carbs: 26 g | Fiber: 11 g | Cholesterol: 221 mg | Sodium: 515 mg | Potassium: 481 mg

Useful Tip: For a heartier option, you can add sautéed spinach or sliced avocado to the burrito filling.

Mango Coconut Breakfast Rice Bowl

Serving: 4 | Prep time: 10 minutes | Cook time: 20 minutes

Ingredients:

- 6.3 oz (180 g) uncooked jasmine rice
- 14 oz (415 ml) coconut milk
- 1 ripe mango, peeled, pitted, and diced
- 1 oz (28 g) unsweetened shredded coconut
- 1 tbsp honey or maple syrup

- 1/4 tsp ground turmeric
- 1/4 tsp ground cinnamon
- Pinch of salt
- Chopped fresh mint leaves (for garnish)

Directions:

1. Rinse the jasmine rice under cold water until the water runs clear.
2. In a medium saucepan, combine the rinsed rice, coconut milk, and a pinch of salt. Bring to a boil, then reduce the heat to low, cover, and simmer for 15-18 minutes, or until the rice is cooked and the liquid is absorbed.
3. In a separate bowl, combine the diced mango, unsweetened shredded coconut, honey or maple syrup, ground turmeric, ground cinnamon, and a pinch of salt. Mix well to coat the mango with the spices and sweetener.
4. Once the rice is cooked, fluff it with a fork and divide it among serving bowls.
5. Top each bowl of rice with the mango coconut mixture.
6. Garnish with chopped fresh mint leaves for a burst of freshness.
7. Serve the mango coconut rice bowl warm.

Nutritional Values: Calories: 250 kcal | Fat: 11 g | Protein: 3 g | Carbs: 37 g | Net carbs: 32 g | Fiber: 5 g | Cholesterol: 0 mg | Sodium: 20 mg | Potassium: 300 mg

Useful Tip: For added crunch and texture, sprinkle chopped toasted almonds or cashews on top of the rice bowl before serving.

Broccoli and Cheese Egg Muffins

Serving: 4 | Prep time: 10 minutes | Cook time: 20 minutes

Ingredients:

- 6 large eggs
- 2 oz (60 ml) milk
- 4 oz (115 g) chopped broccoli florets
- 2 oz (60 g) shredded cheddar cheese
- 1 oz (28 g) diced red bell pepper

- 2 green onions , finely chopped
- 1/4 tsp garlic powder
- Salt and pepper to taste
- Cooking spray or olive oil for greasing
- Fresh chives, chopped (for garnish)

Directions:

1. Preheat the oven to 350°F (175°C) and lightly grease a muffin tin with cooking spray or olive oil.
2. In a mixing bowl, whisk together the eggs and milk until well combined.
3. Stir in the chopped broccoli, shredded cheddar cheese, diced red bell pepper, chopped green onions, garlic powder, salt, and pepper.
4. Pour the egg mixture evenly into the prepared muffin tin, filling each cup about 3/4 full.
5. Bake in the preheated oven for 18-20 minutes, or until the egg muffins are set and slightly golden on top.
6. Remove from the oven and let the muffins cool for a few minutes in the tin before carefully removing them.
7. Garnish with chopped fresh chives for an added burst of flavor.
8. Serve the broccoli and cheese egg muffins warm or at room temperature.

Nutritional Values: Calories: 146 kcal | Fat: 10 g | Protein: 11 g | Carbs: 3 g | Net carbs: 2 g | Fiber: 1 g | Cholesterol: 279 mg | Sodium: 232 mg | Potassium: 209 mg

Useful Tip: These egg muffins can be prepared ahead of time and refrigerated. Simply reheat them in the microwave for a quick and convenient breakfast.

Blueberry Lemon Poppy Seed Muffins

Serving: 4 | Prep time: 15 minutes | Cook time: 20 minutes

Ingredients:

- 6 oz (170 g) almond flour
- 1 oz (28 g) coconut flour
- 2 oz (60 ml) olive oil
- 2 oz (60 ml) unsweetened almond milk
- 3 large eggs
- 1.75 oz (50 g) erythritol (or sweetener of choice)

- 1 tbsp lemon zest
- 2 tbsp lemon juice
- 1 tsp baking powder
- 1/4 tsp salt
- 1 oz (28 g) poppy seeds
- 2.5 oz (70 g) blueberries (fresh or frozen)

Directions:

1. Preheat the oven to 350°F (175°C) and line a muffin tin with parchment paper liners.
2. In a large bowl, whisk together the almond flour, coconut flour, baking powder, and salt.
3. In a separate bowl, whisk together the olive oil, almond milk, eggs, erythritol, lemon zest, and lemon juice until well combined.
4. Add the wet ingredients to the dry ingredients and mix until a batter forms.
5. Stir in the poppy seeds and blueberries until evenly distributed in the batter.
6. Divide the batter evenly among the muffin cups, filling each about 3/4 full.
7. Bake in the preheated oven for 18-20 minutes, or until the muffins are golden and a toothpick inserted into the center comes out clean.
8. Remove from the oven and let the muffins cool in the tin for a few minutes before transferring to a wire rack to cool completely.

Nutritional Values: Calories: 240 kcal | Fat: 20 g | Protein: 8 g | Carbs: 9 g | Net carbs: 4 g | Fiber: 5 g | Cholesterol: 93 mg | Sodium: 222 mg | Potassium: 140 mg

Useful Tip: To ensure even distribution of blueberries, you can toss them in a little coconut flour before adding them to the batter. This helps prevent them from sinking to the bottom during baking.

Greek Yogurt Berry Parfait with Granola

Serving: 4 | Prep time: 10 minutes | Cook time: 0 minutes

Ingredients:

- 16 oz (450 g) plain Greek yogurt
- 8 oz (225 g) mixed berries (strawberries, blueberries, raspberries)
- 2 oz (55 g) granola

- 1 oz (28 g) chopped nuts (almonds, walnuts)
- 1 tbsp honey or maple syrup
- 1 tsp vanilla extract

Directions:

1. In a bowl, mix the Greek yogurt, honey or maple syrup, and vanilla extract until well combined.
2. Wash and prepare the berries as needed, slicing strawberries if desired.
3. In serving glasses or bowls, layer the Greek yogurt mixture, mixed berries, and granola, repeating the layers as desired.
4. Top each parfait with chopped nuts for added crunch and texture.
5. Serve immediately or refrigerate until ready to enjoy.

Nutritional Values: Calories: 280 kcal | Fat: 8 g | Protein: 16 g | Carbs: 40 g | Net carbs: 28 g | Fiber: 12 g | Cholesterol: 10 mg | Sodium: 70 mg | Potassium: 310 mg

Useful Tip: Customize the parfait by using your favorite berries and swapping the nuts for seeds like chia seeds or flaxseeds for an extra nutritional boost.

Caramelized Onion and Spinach Breakfast Casserole

Serving: 4 | Prep time: 15 minutes | Cook time: 40 minutes

Ingredients:

- 8 large eggs
- 8 oz (225 g) baby spinach, chopped
- 1 large onion, thinly sliced
- 4 oz (115 g) feta cheese, crumbled
- 4 oz (115 g) shredded cheddar cheese
- 2 tbsp olive oil
- 1 tbsp butter
- 1/2 tsp salt
- 1/4 tsp black pepper
- 1/4 tsp dried thyme
- 1/4 tsp red pepper flakes (optional)

Directions:

1. Preheat the oven to 350°F (175°C). Grease a baking dish.
2. In a large skillet, heat the olive oil and butter over medium heat. Add the sliced onion and cook, stirring occasionally, until caramelized and golden brown, about 15-20 minutes.
3. Add the chopped spinach to the skillet and sauté until wilted, about 2-3 minutes. Remove from heat and let cool slightly.
4. In a mixing bowl, whisk the eggs until well beaten. Stir in the crumbled feta cheese, shredded cheddar cheese, salt, black pepper, dried thyme, and red pepper flakes if using.
5. Stir in the caramelized onion and spinach mixture into the egg mixture until well combined.
6. Pour the mixture into the prepared baking dish and spread it evenly.
7. Bake in the preheated oven for about 20-25 minutes or until the casserole is set and the top is lightly golden.
8. Let the casserole cool for a few minutes before slicing and serving.

Nutritional Values: Calories: 280 kcal | Fat: 21 g | Protein: 17 g | Carbs: 7 g | Net carbs: 5 g | Fiber: 2 g | Cholesterol: 390 mg | Sodium: 650 mg | Potassium: 470 mg

Useful Tip: Feel free to customize this casserole by adding other vegetables like bell peppers, mushrooms, or tomatoes for added flavor and nutrients.

Avocado and Bacon Breakfast Tacos

Serving: 4 | Prep time: 10 minutes | Cook time: 10 minutes

Ingredients:

- 8 small corn or whole wheat tortillas
- 4 large eggs
- 2 ripe avocados, sliced
- 8 strips cooked bacon, crumbled
- 2 oz (57 g) diced tomatoes
- 1 oz (28 g) diced red onion
- 1 oz (28 g) shredded cheddar cheese
- 2 tbsp olive oil
- Salt and pepper to taste
- Fresh cilantro, chopped (for garnish)
- Hot sauce (optional, for serving)

Directions:

1. Heat the tortillas according to the package instructions and keep them warm.
2. In a skillet, heat 1 tablespoon of olive oil over medium heat.
3. Crack the eggs into the skillet and cook to your preferred doneness (scrambled or fried).
4. While the eggs are cooking, prepare the avocado slices, crumbled bacon, diced tomatoes, and diced red onion.
5. Assemble the tacos: Place a few slices of avocado on each tortilla, followed by the cooked eggs, crumbled bacon, diced tomatoes, and diced red onion.
6. Sprinkle shredded cheddar cheese on top and drizzle with a little more olive oil.
7. Season with salt and pepper to taste and garnish with chopped cilantro.
8. Serve the tacos with hot sauce on the side, if desired.

Nutritional Values: Calories: 318 kcal | Fat: 22 g | Protein: 13 g | Carbs: 20 g | Net carbs: 14 g | Fiber: 6 g | Cholesterol: 189 mg | Sodium: 449 mg | Potassium: 577 mg

Useful Tip: Customize these tacos with your favorite toppings, such as diced bell peppers, sautéed mushrooms, or a squeeze of lime juice for added flavor.

Poultry Recipes

Herb-Roasted Chicken with Garlic Mashed Cauliflower

Serving: 4 | Prep time: 15 minutes | Cook time: 35 minutes

Ingredients:

For the Herb-Roasted Chicken:

- 4 boneless, skinless chicken breasts
- 2 tbsp olive oil
- 1 tsp dried thyme
- 1 tsp dried rosemary
- 1 tsp dried oregano
- Salt and pepper to taste

For the Garlic Mashed Cauliflower:

- 1 medium head cauliflower, cut into florets
- 3 cloves garlic, minced
- 2 tbsp butter
- 2 oz (60 ml) unsweetened almond milk
- Salt and pepper to taste

For Garnish:

- Fresh chopped parsley

Directions:

1. Preheat the oven to 400°F (200°C).
2. In a small bowl, mix together the dried thyme, rosemary, oregano, salt, and pepper.
3. Place the chicken breasts on a baking sheet lined with parchment paper. Brush each chicken breast with olive oil and then sprinkle the herb mixture evenly over both sides of the chicken.
4. Roast the chicken in the preheated oven for about 25-30 minutes, or until the internal temperature reaches 165°F (74°C) and the chicken is cooked through.
5. While the chicken is roasting, prepare the garlic mashed cauliflower. Steam the cauliflower florets until they are tender, about 10-12 minutes.
6. In a saucepan, melt the butter over medium heat. Add the minced garlic and sauté for about 1 minute until fragrant.
7. Remove the saucepan from the heat and add the steamed cauliflower, almond milk, salt, and pepper. Mash the cauliflower with a potato masher until it reaches your desired consistency.
8. Serve the herb-roasted chicken over a bed of garlic mashed cauliflower. Garnish with fresh chopped parsley.

Nutritional Values: Calories: 250 kcal | Fat: 12 g | Protein: 28 g | Carbs: 9 g | Net carbs: 6 g | Fiber: 3 g | Cholesterol: 75 mg | Sodium: 250 mg | Potassium: 800 mg

Useful Tip: You can customize the herb mixture for the chicken with your favorite herbs and spices to suit your taste preferences.

Lemon Thyme Grilled Turkey Cutlets with Zucchini Noodles

Serving: 4 | Prep time: 20 minutes | Cook time: 15 minutes

Ingredients:

- 16 oz (450 g) turkey cutlets
- 3 medium zucchinis, spiralized into noodles
- 2 tbsp olive oil
- 2 tbsp fresh lemon juice
- 2 tsp lemon zest
- 2 tsp fresh thyme leaves
- Salt and pepper to taste
- 2 cloves garlic, minced
- 1/4 tsp red pepper flakes
- 2 oz (60 ml) low-sodium chicken broth
- 1 tbsp grated Parmesan cheese
- Fresh thyme sprigs for garnish

Directions:

1. Marinate the turkey cutlets in olive oil, lemon juice, lemon zest, fresh thyme leaves, minced garlic, salt, and pepper for 15 minutes.
2. Preheat your grill or grill pan to medium-high heat, then grill the turkey cutlets for 4-5 minutes on each side until fully cooked and grill marks form.
3. Sauté spiralized zucchini noodles and red pepper flakes in a skillet over medium heat for 2-3 minutes until noodles are tender.
4. Pour in the chicken broth and cook for an additional 1-2 minutes to infuse flavors.
5. Remove zucchini noodles from heat, toss with grated Parmesan cheese, and season with salt and pepper if desired.
6. Serve by placing zucchini noodles on plates, topping with grilled turkey cutlets, and garnishing with fresh thyme sprigs.
7. Enjoy the dish.

Nutritional Values: Calories: 290 kcal | Fat: 12 g | Protein: 34 g | Carbs: 12 g | Net carbs: 8 g | Fiber: 4 g | Cholesterol: 95 mg | Sodium: 230 mg | Potassium: 830 mg

Useful Tip: To enhance the lemony flavor, consider marinating the turkey cutlets for a few hours or overnight for an even more vibrant taste.

Sesame Ginger Glazed Chicken Skewers with Cauliflower Rice

Serving: 4 | Prep time: 25 minutes | Cook time: 15 minutes

Ingredients:

- 1 lb (450 g) boneless, skinless chicken breasts, cut into bite-sized pieces
- 2 tbsp low-sodium soy sauce
- 1 tbsp sesame oil
- 1 tbsp rice vinegar
- 2 tsp grated fresh ginger
- 2 cloves garlic, minced
- 1 tbsp honey
- 1 tbsp water
- 2 tsp sesame seeds
- Salt and pepper to taste
- 1 medium cauliflower, riced
- 2 green onions, chopped
- 1 tbsp olive oil
- Lime wedges for serving

Directions:

1. In a bowl, whisk together soy sauce, sesame oil, rice vinegar, grated ginger, minced garlic, honey, water, sesame seeds, salt, and pepper to create the marinade.
2. Place the chicken pieces in a resealable bag and pour half of the marinade over them. Seal the bag and marinate in the refrigerator for at least 15 minutes.
3. While the chicken is marinating, prepare the cauliflower rice by pulsing the cauliflower florets in a food processor until they resemble rice grains.
4. Heat olive oil in a skillet over medium heat, add the riced cauliflower, and sauté for about 5-6 minutes until tender.
5. Thread the marinated chicken pieces onto skewers and grill or cook on a grill pan over medium-high heat for about 6-8 minutes, turning occasionally, until cooked through and slightly charred.
6. Warm the remaining marinade in a small saucepan until slightly thickened.
7. Serve the grilled chicken skewers over a bed of cauliflower rice, drizzle with the warmed marinade, and sprinkle with chopped green onions. Serve with lime wedges.
8. Enjoy the dish.

Nutritional Values: Calories: 280 kcal | Fat: 10 g | Protein: 32 g | Carbs: 15 g | Net carbs: 10 g | Fiber: 5 g | Cholesterol: 75 mg | Sodium: 430 mg | Potassium: 800 mg

Useful Tip: Soak wooden skewers in water for about 15 minutes before threading the chicken to prevent them from burning during grilling.

Spiced Paprika Chicken Thighs with Roasted Brussels Sprouts

Serving: 4 | Prep time: 15 minutes | Cook time: 25 minutes

Ingredients:

- 4 bone-in, skin-on chicken thighs
- 2 tbsp olive oil
- 2 tsp paprika
- 1 tsp ground cumin
- 1/2 tsp ground coriander
- 1/2 tsp garlic powder
- Salt and pepper to taste
- 1 lb (450 g) Brussels sprouts, trimmed and halved
- 1 tbsp balsamic vinegar
- Fresh parsley, chopped, for garnish
- Lemon wedges for serving

Directions:

1. Preheat the oven to 425°F (220°C).
2. In a bowl, mix together olive oil, paprika, ground cumin, ground coriander, garlic powder, salt, and pepper to create the spice rub.
3. Pat the chicken thighs dry and rub the spice mixture all over the chicken, ensuring it's well coated.
4. Place the chicken thighs, skin side up, on a baking sheet lined with parchment paper.
5. Toss the Brussels sprouts with balsamic vinegar and a drizzle of olive oil on another baking sheet.
6. Roast both the chicken and Brussels sprouts in the preheated oven for about 20-25 minutes or until the chicken is cooked through and the Brussels sprouts are crispy and tender.
7. Transfer the chicken and Brussels sprouts to serving plates, garnish with chopped parsley, and serve with lemon wedges on the side.
8. **Enjoy the dish.**

Nutritional Values: Calories: 360 kcal | Fat: 22 g | Protein: 28 g | Carbs: 15 g | Net carbs: 10 g | Fiber: 5 g | Cholesterol: 140 mg | Sodium: 320 mg | Potassium: 970 mg

Useful Tip: For extra crispy Brussels sprouts, make sure they are spread out in a single layer on the baking sheet and avoid crowding them. This allows them to roast evenly and develop that delicious caramelized texture.

Orange Rosemary Baked Quail with Sautéed Spinach

Serving: 4 | Prep time: 20 minutes | Cook time: 30 minutes

Ingredients:

- 4 whole quail, cleaned and patted dry
- 2 oranges, zested and juiced
- 2 tbsp olive oil
- 2 tsp fresh rosemary, finely chopped
- Salt and pepper to taste
- 1 lb (450 g) fresh spinach leaves
- 2 cloves garlic, minced
- 1 tbsp lemon juice
- Lemon wedges for serving

Directions:

1. Preheat the oven to 375°F (190°C).
2. In a bowl, mix together orange zest, orange juice, olive oil, chopped rosemary, salt, and pepper.
3. Rub the mixture all over the quail, ensuring they're well coated.
4. Place the quail in a baking dish and bake in the preheated oven for about 25-30 minutes or until the quail are cooked through and golden.
5. While the quail are baking, heat a skillet over medium heat and add a drizzle of olive oil.
6. Sauté the minced garlic until fragrant, then add the fresh spinach leaves and cook until wilted.
7. Drizzle lemon juice over the sautéed spinach and season with salt and pepper.
8. Serve the baked quail over a bed of sautéed spinach, accompanied by lemon wedges for an extra burst of flavor.
9. Enjoy the dish.

Nutritional Values: Calories: 320 kcal | Fat: 18 g | Protein: 32 g | Carbs: 12 g | Net carbs: 8 g | Fiber: 4 g | Cholesterol: 120 mg | Sodium: 220 mg | Potassium: 1000 mg

Useful Tip: To make the quail even more flavorful, consider marinating them in the orange-rosemary mixture for an hour before baking – this will infuse the meat with the vibrant citrus and herb notes.

Crispy Dijon Mustard Chicken Tenders with Roasted Asparagus

Serving: 4 | Prep time: 15 minutes | Cook time: 20 minutes

Ingredients:

- 1 lb (450 g) chicken tenders
- 2 oz (63 g) Dijon mustard
- 2 tbsp olive oil
- 1 tsp garlic powder
- 1 tsp dried thyme
- Salt and pepper to taste
- 1 lb (450 g) asparagus spears, trimmed
- 1 tbsp balsamic vinegar
- Fresh parsley, chopped, for garnish
- Lemon wedges for serving

Directions:

1. Preheat the oven to 425°F (220°C).
2. In a bowl, mix together Dijon mustard, olive oil, garlic powder, dried thyme, salt, and pepper.
3. Coat each chicken tender with the Dijon mustard mixture, ensuring they're well coated.
4. Place the chicken tenders on a baking sheet lined with parchment paper and bake in the preheated oven for about 15-20 minutes or until the chicken is cooked through and crispy.
5. While the chicken is baking, toss the trimmed asparagus with balsamic vinegar and a drizzle of olive oil.
6. Arrange the asparagus on another baking sheet and roast in the oven for about 10-12 minutes until tender.
7. Serve the crispy Dijon mustard chicken tenders alongside roasted asparagus, garnished with chopped parsley and accompanied by lemon wedges.
8. **Enjoy the dish.**

Nutritional Values: Calories: 310 kcal | Fat: 15 g | Protein: 35 g | Carbs: 10 g | Net carbs: 6 g | Fiber: 4 g | Cholesterol: 85 mg | Sodium: 390 mg | Potassium: 750 mg

Useful Tip: For an extra crispy texture, you can briefly broil the chicken tenders for the last 1-2 minutes of cooking, keeping a close eye to prevent over-browning. This will give the chicken an irresistible crunch.

Coconut Curry Chicken Stir-Fry with Cauliflower Rice

Serving: 4 | Prep time: 20 minutes | Cook time: 15 minutes

Ingredients:

- 1 lb (450 g) boneless, skinless chicken breasts, thinly sliced
- 2 tbsp coconut oil
- 1 onion, thinly sliced
- 1 red bell pepper, thinly sliced
- 5 oz (200 g) broccoli florets
- 3 oz (100 g) snap peas, trimmed
- 1 can (13.5 oz / 400 ml) coconut milk
- 2 tbsp red curry paste
- 1 tbsp fish sauce
- 1 tsp ground turmeric
- Salt and pepper to taste
- 1 small head cauliflower, riced
- Fresh cilantro, chopped, for garnish
- Lime wedges for serving

Directions:

1. In a wok or large skillet, heat coconut oil over medium-high heat.
2. Add sliced chicken and stir-fry until cooked through and lightly browned. Remove from the wok and set aside.
3. In the same wok, add sliced onion, red bell pepper, broccoli florets, and snap peas. Stir-fry for about 3-4 minutes until vegetables are crisp-tender.
4. Push the vegetables to one side of the wok and add red curry paste. Stir-fry the paste for about 1 minute until fragrant.
5. Pour in the coconut milk, fish sauce, ground turmeric, salt, and pepper. Stir to combine the curry paste and coconut milk.
6. Return the cooked chicken to the wok and simmer for about 5 minutes until the flavors meld together.
7. While the curry is simmering, rice the cauliflower by pulsing it in a food processor until it resembles rice grains.
8. In a separate pan, sauté the riced cauliflower in a little coconut oil until tender.
9. Serve the coconut curry chicken stir-fry over cauliflower rice, garnished with chopped cilantro and lime wedges on the side.
10. Enjoy the dish.

Nutritional Values: Calories: 380 kcal | Fat: 23 g | Protein: 28 g | Carbs: 18 g | Net carbs: 13 g | Fiber: 5 g | Cholesterol: 70 mg | Sodium: 650 mg | Potassium: 900 mg

Useful Tip: For a creamier curry, you can opt for full-fat coconut milk, but for a lighter version, choose light coconut milk to reduce the calorie and fat content.

Honey Sriracha Glazed Turkey Meatballs with Steamed Broccoli

Serving: 4 | Prep time: 25 minutes | Cook time: 20 minutes

Ingredients:

- 1 lb (450 g) ground turkey
- 1 oz (60 ml) breadcrumbs
- 1 egg
- 2 cloves garlic, minced
- 1 tsp grated ginger
- 2 oz (60 ml) honey
- 2 tbsp Sriracha sauce
- 1 tbsp soy sauce
- Salt and pepper to taste
- 1 lb (450 g) broccoli florets
- Sesame seeds for garnish
- Green onions, sliced, for garnish

Directions:

1. Preheat the oven to 375°F (190°C).
2. In a bowl, mix together ground turkey, breadcrumbs, egg, minced garlic, grated ginger, salt, and pepper.
3. Form the mixture into meatballs and place them on a baking sheet lined with parchment paper.
4. Bake the meatballs in the preheated oven for about 15-20 minutes or until cooked through and lightly browned.
5. In a small saucepan, combine honey, Sriracha sauce, and soy sauce. Heat over low heat until the mixture is well combined and slightly thickened.
6. Toss the baked meatballs in the honey Sriracha glaze until coated.
7. While the meatballs are baking, steam the broccoli florets until they are tender, about 5-7 minutes.
8. Serve the honey Sriracha glazed turkey meatballs alongside steamed broccoli, and garnish with sesame seeds and sliced green onions.
9. **Enjoy the dish.**

Nutritional Values: Calories: 320 kcal | Fat: 12 g | Protein: 28 g | Carbs: 28 g | Net carbs: 24 g | Fiber: 4 g | Cholesterol: 100 mg | Sodium: 800 mg | Potassium: 900 mg

Useful Tip: If you prefer a milder flavor, you can adjust the Sriracha sauce quantity in the glaze to suit your taste preferences.

Mango Chipotle Grilled Chicken Breast with Cilantro Lime Cauliflower Rice

Serving: 4 | Prep time: 25 minutes | Cook time: 20 minutes

Ingredients:

- 4 boneless, skinless chicken breasts
- 1 ripe mango, peeled and pitted
- 1 chipotle pepper in adobo sauce
- 2 tbsp olive oil
- Juice of 1 lime
- Salt and pepper to taste
- 1 medium head cauliflower, riced
- 1 oz (15 g) fresh cilantro, chopped
- Lime wedges for serving

Directions:

1. In a blender, combine the mango, chipotle pepper, olive oil, lime juice, salt, and pepper. Blend until smooth to make the marinade.
2. Place the chicken breasts in a resealable bag and pour the mango chipotle marinade over them. Seal the bag and marinate in the refrigerator for at least 15 minutes.
3. Preheat the grill to medium-high heat.
4. Remove the chicken breasts from the marinade and grill them for about 6-8 minutes on each side or until they are cooked through and have nice grill marks.
5. While the chicken is grilling, rice the cauliflower by pulsing it in a food processor until it resembles rice grains.
6. In a skillet, sauté the riced cauliflower over medium heat for about 4-5 minutes until tender.
7. Stir in the chopped cilantro and lime juice, and season with salt and pepper.
8. Serve the grilled mango chipotle chicken breast over a bed of cilantro lime cauliflower rice, and garnish with lime wedges.
9. Enjoy the dish.

Nutritional Values: Calories: 320 kcal | Fat: 10 g | Protein: 35 g | Carbs: 25 g | Net carbs: 19 g | Fiber: 6 g | Cholesterol: 85 mg | Sodium: 320 mg | Potassium: 850 mg

Useful Tip: For a sweeter marinade, you can add a touch of honey or maple syrup to balance the heat from the chipotle pepper, creating a perfect sweet and spicy combination.

Garlic Parmesan Crusted Chicken with Roasted Carrots

Serving: 4 | Prep time: 20 minutes | Cook time: 25 minutes

Ingredients:

- 4 boneless, skinless chicken breasts
- 1 oz (50 g) grated Parmesan cheese
- 1 oz (30 g) almond flour
- 2 cloves garlic, minced
- 1 tsp dried oregano
- Salt and pepper to taste
- 2 tbsp olive oil
- 1 lb (450 g) carrots, peeled and cut into sticks
- 1 tbsp balsamic vinegar
- Fresh parsley, chopped, for garnish
- Lemon wedges for serving

Directions:

1. Preheat the oven to 400°F (200°C).
2. In a bowl, mix together grated Parmesan cheese, almond flour, minced garlic, dried oregano, salt, and pepper.
3. Pat the chicken breasts dry and coat them with the Parmesan mixture, pressing it onto the chicken to adhere.
4. In a skillet, heat olive oil over medium-high heat.
5. Add the coated chicken breasts and cook for about 3-4 minutes on each side until golden brown.
6. Transfer the chicken to a baking dish and finish cooking in the preheated oven for about 15-20 minutes or until the chicken is cooked through.
7. While the chicken is baking, toss the carrot sticks with balsamic vinegar and a drizzle of olive oil.
8. Arrange the carrots on a baking sheet and roast in the oven for about 15 minutes until tender.
9. Serve the garlic Parmesan crusted chicken alongside roasted carrots, garnished with chopped parsley and accompanied by lemon wedges.
10. Enjoy the dish.

Nutritional Values: Calories: 380 kcal | Fat: 18 g | Protein: 40 g | Carbs: 20 g | Net carbs: 14 g | Fiber: 6 g | Cholesterol: 100 mg | Sodium: 480 mg | Potassium: 1050 mg

Useful Tip: For an extra crispy crust on the chicken, you can briefly broil it for the last 1-2 minutes of baking, watching closely to prevent over-browning.

Meat Recipes

Tender Herb-Marinated Pork Chops with Lemon Herb Green Beans

Serving: 4 | Prep time: 15 minutes | Cook time: 20 minutes

Ingredients:

- 4 boneless pork chops
- 2 oz (60 ml) olive oil
- 2 cloves garlic, minced
- 2 tbsp fresh parsley, chopped
- 1 tbsp fresh thyme leaves
- Salt and pepper, to taste
- 1 lb (450 g) fresh green beans, trimmed
- Zest and juice of 1 lemon
- 2 tbsp olive oil
- Salt and pepper, to taste

Directions:

1. In a bowl, whisk together 2 oz (60 ml) of olive oil, minced garlic, chopped parsley, fresh thyme leaves, salt, and pepper to create the herb marinade.
2. Pat the pork chops dry and place them in a resealable bag. Pour the herb marinade over the pork chops, seal the bag, and massage the marinade into the meat. Allow to marinate for at least 15 minutes.
3. Preheat a skillet or grill over medium-high heat.
4. Remove the pork chops from the marinade, allowing any excess to drip off. Cook the pork chops for about 4-5 minutes on each side, or until the internal temperature reaches 145°F (63°C) and the meat is no longer pink in the center.
5. While the pork chops are cooking, blanch the green beans in boiling water for about 2 minutes until they're bright green and slightly tender. Drain and set aside.
6. In a bowl, whisk together the lemon zest, lemon juice, 2 tablespoons of olive oil, salt, and pepper to create the lemon herb dressing.
7. Toss the blanched green beans in the lemon herb dressing until they're well coated.
8. Serve the tender herb-marinated pork chops alongside the lemon herb green beans.
9. Enjoy the dish.

Nutritional Values: Calories: 360 kcal | Fat: 20 g | Protein: 35 g | Carbs: 12 g | Net carbs: 8 g | Fiber: 4 g | Cholesterol: 90 mg | Sodium: 100 mg | Potassium: 950 mg

Useful Tip: Allow the pork chops to rest for a few minutes after cooking to lock in their juices before serving.

Spiced Lamb Meatballs with Cumin-Scented Cauliflower Rice

Serving: 4 | Prep time: 20 minutes | Cook time: 25 minutes

Ingredients:

For the Lamb Meatballs:

- 1 lb (450 g) ground lamb
- 1 oz (25 g) finely chopped onion
- 2 cloves garlic, minced
- 1 tsp ground cumin
- 1/2 tsp ground coriander
- 1/2 tsp smoked paprika
- 1/4 tsp cayenne pepper
- Salt and pepper to taste
- 1 tbsp olive oil, for cooking

For the Cumin-Scented Cauliflower Rice:

- 1 medium head cauliflower, riced
- 1 tbsp olive oil
- 1 tsp ground cumin
- Salt and pepper to taste
- Fresh cilantro leaves, chopped,for Garnish:
- Lemon wedges, for serving:

Directions:

1. In a mixing bowl, combine the ground lamb, chopped onion, minced garlic, ground cumin, ground coriander, smoked paprika, cayenne pepper, salt, and pepper. Mix well until all the spices are evenly distributed.
2. Shape the mixture into meatballs, approximately 1.5 inches in diameter.
3. In a large skillet, heat the olive oil over medium-high heat. Add the lamb meatballs and cook until browned on all sides and cooked through, about 8-10 minutes. Remove the meatballs from the skillet and set them aside.
4. In the same skillet, add another tablespoon of olive oil and heat over medium heat. Add the riced cauliflower, ground cumin, salt, and pepper. Cook, stirring occasionally, until the cauliflower rice is tender and lightly golden, about 5-7 minutes.
5. To serve, divide the cumin-scented cauliflower rice among plates, top with spiced lamb meatballs, and garnish with chopped cilantro. Serve with lemon wedges on the side.

Nutritional Values: Calories: 385 kcal | Fat: 28 g | Protein: 24 g | Carbs: 10 g | Net carbs: 7 g | Fiber: 3 g | Cholesterol: 93 mg | Sodium: 125 mg | Potassium: 763 mg

Useful Tip: For a richer flavor, you can sauté the cauliflower rice with finely chopped garlic and diced onion before adding the ground cumin.

Savory Rosemary Roast Beef with Sautéed Mushrooms and Asparagus

Serving: 4 | Prep time: 15 minutes | Cook time: 40 minutes

Ingredients:

For the Roast Beef:

- 1.5 lb (680 g) beef roast (such as sirloin or tenderloin)
- 2 tbsp olive oil
- 2 tsp fresh rosemary, minced
- Salt and pepper to taste

For the Sautéed Mushrooms:

- 8 oz (225 g) mushrooms, sliced
- 2 cloves garlic, minced
- 2 tbsp butter
- Salt and pepper to taste

For the Asparagus:

- 1 bunch asparagus, tough ends trimmed
- 2 tbsp olive oil
- Salt and pepper to taste

Directions:

1. Preheat the oven to 375°F (190°C).
2. In a small bowl, combine the olive oil, minced rosemary, salt, and pepper. Rub this mixture all over the beef roast.
3. Place the seasoned beef roast on a roasting pan or oven-safe skillet. Roast in the preheated oven for about 25-30 minutes, or until the internal temperature reaches your desired level of doneness (145°F / 63°C for medium-rare, 160°F / 71°C for medium). Remove the roast from the oven and let it rest for 10 minutes before slicing.
4. While the roast is resting, prepare the sautéed mushrooms. In a skillet over medium heat, melt the butter. Add the sliced mushrooms and minced garlic, then sauté until the mushrooms are tender and golden, about 5-7 minutes. Season with salt and pepper.
5. For the asparagus, preheat another skillet over medium-high heat. Add olive oil and swirl to coat the pan. Add the trimmed asparagus and sauté until tender-crisp, about 4-5 minutes. Season with salt and pepper.

Nutritional Values: Calories: 350 kcal | Fat: 20 g | Protein: 35 g | Carbs: 6 g | Net carbs: 4 g | Fiber: 2 g | Cholesterol: 100 mg | Sodium: 150 mg | Potassium: 800 mg

Useful Tip: To add an extra layer of flavor to the roast beef, marinate it in the rosemary-olive oil mixture for an hour before cooking.

Chimichurri Marinated Grilled Pork Tenderloin with Roasted Brussels Sprouts

Serving: 4 | Prep time: 20 minutes | Cook time: 25 minutes

Ingredients:

For the Pork Tenderloin:

- 1 lb (450 g) pork tenderloin
- 4 oz (118 ml) chimichurri sauce (homemade or
- store-bought)
- Salt and pepper to taste

For the Roasted Brussels Sprouts:

- 1 lb (450 g) Brussels sprouts, trimmed and halved
- 2 tbsp olive oil
- Salt and pepper to taste

Directions:

1. Preheat the grill to medium-high heat.
2. Place the pork tenderloin in a zip-top bag or shallow dish and pour the chimichurri sauce over it. Make sure the pork is coated with the sauce. Marinate for at least 15 minutes, or up to 2 hours in the refrigerator.
3. While the pork is marinating, preheat the oven to 400°F (200°C).
4. In a bowl, toss the halved Brussels sprouts with olive oil, salt, and pepper until well coated. Spread them in a single layer on a baking sheet.
5. Roast the Brussels sprouts in the preheated oven for 20-25 minutes, or until they are tender and nicely browned, stirring halfway through.
6. Grill the marinated pork tenderloin on the preheated grill for about 6-8 minutes per side, or until the internal temperature reaches 145°F (63°C) for medium-rare, or up to 160°F (71°C) for medium, depending on your preference.
7. Once the pork is cooked, remove it from the grill and let it rest for a few minutes before slicing.

Nutritional Values: Calories: 300 kcal | Fat: 12 g | Protein: 30 g | Carbs: 18 g | Net carbs: 10 g | Fiber: 8 g | Cholesterol: 75 mg | Sodium: 300 mg | Potassium: 900 mg

Useful Tip: For an extra burst of flavor, brush some of the chimichurri sauce over the grilled pork tenderloin just before taking it off the grill.

Tender Ginger-Soy Marinated Beef Stir-Fry with Cauliflower Rice

Serving: 4 | Prep time: 15 minutes | Cook time: 15 minutes

Ingredients:

For the Beef Marinade:

- 1 lb (450 g) beef sirloin, thinly sliced
- 2 tbsp low-sodium soy sauce
- 1 tbsp fresh ginger, minced
- 2 cloves garlic, minced

- 1 tbsp sesame oil
- 1 tbsp rice vinegar
- 1 tsp honey or a low-carb sweetener
- 1 tsp cornstarch (optional, for thickening)

For the Stir-Fry:

- 2 tbsp vegetable oil, divided
- 1 red bell pepper, thinly sliced
- 6 oz (175 g) broccoli florets

- 5 oz (150 g) snap peas, ends trimmed
- Salt and pepper to taste

For the Cauliflower Rice:

- 1 medium head cauliflower, riced
- 2 tbsp vegetable oil

- Salt to taste

Directions:

1. In a bowl, whisk together the soy sauce, minced ginger, minced garlic, sesame oil, rice vinegar, honey (or sweetener), and cornstarch (if using) to create the marinade. Add the sliced beef and toss to coat. Let it marinate for 10-15 minutes.
2. While the beef is marinating, prepare the cauliflower rice. In a large skillet, heat 2 tablespoons of vegetable oil over medium heat. Add the riced cauliflower and cook for 5-7 minutes, stirring occasionally, until the cauliflower is tender. Season with salt to taste.
3. In a separate large skillet or wok, heat 1 tablespoon of vegetable oil over high heat. Add the marinated beef and stir-fry for 2-3 minutes until cooked. Remove the beef from the skillet and set it aside.
4. In the same skillet, add the remaining tablespoon of vegetable oil. Stir-fry the red bell pepper, broccoli florets, and snap peas for 3-4 minutes until they are crisp-tender.
5. Return the cooked beef to the skillet with the vegetables, and stir to combine. Adjust the seasoning with salt and pepper if needed.

Nutritional Values: Calories: 320 kcal | Fat: 18 g | Protein: 25 g | Carbs: 16 g | Net carbs: 10 g | Fiber: 6 g | Cholesterol: 65 mg | Sodium: 500 mg | Potassium: 1000 mg

Useful Tip: To reduce the sodium content, you can use low-sodium soy sauce and adjust the amount of salt in the dish.

Balsamic Glazed Lamb Meatballs with Mediterranean Roasted Eggplant

Serving: 4 | Prep time: 25 minutes | Cook time: 30 minutes

Ingredients:

For the Lamb Meatballs:

- 1 lb (450 g) ground lamb
- 2 oz (23 g) breadcrumbs
- 2 oz (62 g) finely grated Parmesan cheese
- 1 egg

- 2 cloves garlic, minced
- 1 tsp dried oregano
- Salt and pepper to taste
- 1 tbsp olive oil, for cooking

For the Balsamic Glaze:

- 2 oz (60 g) balsamic vinegar

- 2 tbsp honey or a low-carb sweetener

For the Roasted Eggplant:

- 1 large eggplant, cut into 1-inch cubes
- 2 tbsp olive oil

- 1 tsp dried thyme
- Salt and pepper to taste

Directions:

1. Preheat the oven to 400°F (200°C).
2. In a mixing bowl, combine the ground lamb, breadcrumbs, grated Parmesan cheese, egg, minced garlic, dried oregano, salt, and pepper. Mix until well combined.

3. Shape the lamb mixture into meatballs, about 1.5 inches in diameter.
4. Heat the olive oil in an oven-safe skillet over medium-high heat. Add the lamb meatballs and brown them on all sides, about 5-6 minutes. Transfer the skillet to the preheated oven and bake for an additional 10-12 minutes, until the meatballs are cooked through.
5. While the meatballs are baking, prepare the balsamic glaze. In a small saucepan, combine the balsamic vinegar and honey. Bring to a simmer over medium heat and cook for 3-4 minutes, until the mixture thickens. Remove from heat.
6. In a separate baking sheet, toss the eggplant cubes with olive oil, dried thyme, salt, and pepper. Roast in the preheated oven for about 15-20 minutes, until the eggplant is tender and slightly caramelized.

Nutritional Values: Calories: 390 kcal | Fat: 25 g | Protein: 25 g | Carbs: 20 g | Net carbs: 16 g | Fiber: 4 g | Cholesterol: 95 mg | Sodium: 420 mg | Potassium: 700 mg

Useful Tip: For a smoky twist, you can sprinkle a pinch of smoked paprika over the roasted eggplant before baking.

Spiced Paprika Pork Skewers with Zucchini and Red Pepper Medley

Serving: 4 | Prep time: 20 minutes | Cook time: 15 minutes

Ingredients:

For the Pork Skewers:

- 1 lb (450 g) pork loin, cut into 1-inch cubes
- 1 tbsp smoked paprika
- 1 tsp ground cumin
- 1/2 tsp garlic powder
- Salt and pepper to taste
- 2 tbsp olive oil
- Wooden skewers, soaked in water

For the Zucchini and Red Pepper Medley:

- 2 medium zucchinis, sliced into rounds
- 1 red bell pepper, sliced
- 1 tbsp olive oil
- 1 tsp dried oregano
- Salt and pepper to taste

Directions:

1. Preheat the grill or grill pan over medium-high heat.
2. In a bowl, combine the smoked paprika, ground cumin, garlic powder, salt, and pepper. Add the pork cubes and toss them in the spice mixture until well coated.
3. Thread the marinated pork cubes onto the soaked wooden skewers.
4. Drizzle the pork skewers with olive oil and grill them for about 3-4 minutes per side, or until they are cooked through and have nice grill marks.
5. While the pork is grilling, prepare the zucchini and red pepper medley. In a bowl, toss the sliced zucchini and red bell pepper with olive oil, dried oregano, salt, and pepper.
6. Heat a skillet or grill pan over medium heat and add the zucchini and red pepper mixture. Cook for about 5-6 minutes, stirring occasionally, until the vegetables are tender and slightly caramelized.

Nutritional Values: Calories: 320 kcal | Fat: 18 g | Protein: 25 g | Carbs: 14 g | Net carbs: 10 g | Fiber: 4 g | Cholesterol: 75 mg | Sodium: 350 mg | Potassium: 950 mg

Useful Tip: For extra tenderness, you can marinate the pork cubes in the spice mixture for up to an hour before threading them onto skewers.

Cumin-Spiced Grilled Beef Steak with Turmeric Cauliflower Mash

Serving: 4 | Prep time: 15 minutes | Cook time: 20 minutes

Ingredients:

For the Grilled Beef Steak:

- 1.5 lbs (680 g) beef steak (such as sirloin or ribeye)
- 1 tbsp ground cumin
- 1 tsp paprika
- 1/2 tsp ground coriander
- Salt and pepper to taste
- 1 tbsp olive oil

For the Turmeric Cauliflower Mash:

- 1 medium head cauliflower, cut into florets
- 1 tsp ground turmeric
- 2 cloves garlic, minced
- 2 tbsp unsalted butter
- Salt and pepper to taste

Directions:

1. Preheat the grill to medium-high heat.
2. In a small bowl, combine the ground cumin, paprika, ground coriander, salt, and pepper. Rub this spice mixture over the beef steak.
3. Drizzle olive oil over the seasoned steak and let it marinate for about 10-15 minutes while you prepare the cauliflower mash.
4. Steam or boil the cauliflower florets until they are tender. Drain well.
5. In a food processor, blend the cooked cauliflower, ground turmeric, minced garlic, and unsalted butter until smooth and creamy. Season with salt and pepper to taste.
6. Grill the marinated beef steak for about 4-5 minutes per side, or until the desired level of doneness is achieved (145°F / 63°C for medium-rare, 160°F / 71°C for medium). Remove from the grill and let it rest for a few minutes before slicing.

Nutritional Values: Calories: 350 kcal | Fat: 20 g | Protein: 35 g | Carbs: 10 g | Net carbs: 6 g | Fiber: 4 g | Cholesterol: 90 mg | Sodium: 450 mg | Potassium: 900 mg

Useful Tip: To enhance the flavor of the cauliflower mash, you can add a splash of almond milk or chicken broth while blending.

Honey Mustard Glazed Pork Ribs with Garlic Mashed Cauliflower

Serving: 4 | Prep time: 20 minutes | Cook time: 1 hour 15 minutes

Ingredients:

For the Pork Ribs:

- 2 lbs (900 g) pork ribs, cut into individual ribs
- Salt and pepper to taste
- 2 oz (63 g) Dijon mustard
- 2 tbsp honey
- 1 tbsp apple cider vinegar
- 1 tsp smoked paprika

For the Garlic Mashed Cauliflower:

- 1 medium head cauliflower, cut into florets
- 2 cloves garlic, minced
- 2 tbsp unsalted butter
- Salt and pepper to taste

Directions:

1. Preheat the oven to 300°F (150°C).
2. Season the pork ribs with salt and pepper.
3. In a bowl, whisk together the Dijon mustard, honey, apple cider vinegar, and smoked paprika to create the glaze.
4. Brush the glaze over the pork ribs, coating them evenly.
5. Place the glazed ribs on a baking sheet lined with aluminum foil and bake in the preheated oven for about 1 hour, basting occasionally with the glaze.
6. While the ribs are baking, steam or boil the cauliflower florets until they are tender. Drain well.
7. In a food processor, blend the cooked cauliflower, minced garlic, and unsalted butter until smooth and creamy. Season with salt and pepper to taste.
8. Once the ribs are tender and glazed, you can choose to finish them on a hot grill or under the broiler for a few minutes to achieve a caramelized finish.

Nutritional Values: Calories: 450 kcal | Fat: 30 g | Protein: 25 g | Carbs: 20 g | Net carbs: 15 g | Fiber: 5 g | Cholesterol: 85 mg | Sodium: 450 mg | Potassium: 800 mg

Useful Tip: For a richer flavor, you can marinate the pork ribs in the honey mustard glaze for a couple of hours before baking.

Chipotle-Marinated Grilled Beef Sirloin with Smoky Paprika Sweet Potatoes

Serving: 4 | Prep time: 20 minutes | Cook time: 25 minutes

Ingredients:

For the Grilled Beef Sirloin:

- 1.5 lbs (680 g) beef sirloin steak
- 2 chipotle peppers in adobo sauce, minced
- 2 cloves garlic, minced
- 2 tbsp olive oil
- 1 tsp ground cumin
- Salt and pepper to taste

For the Smoky Paprika Sweet Potatoes:

- 2 large sweet potatoes, peeled and cut into 1-inch cubes
- 2 tbsp olive oil
- 1 tsp smoked paprika
- 1/2 tsp ground cumin
- Salt and pepper to taste

Directions:

1. Preheat the grill to medium-high heat.
2. In a bowl, combine the minced chipotle peppers, minced garlic, olive oil, ground cumin, salt, and pepper to create the marinade.
3. Rub the marinade over the beef sirloin steak, making sure it is evenly coated. Let it marinate for at least 15 minutes.
4. While the beef is marinating, preheat the oven to 400°F (200°C).
5. In a large bowl, toss the sweet potato cubes with olive oil, smoked paprika, ground cumin, salt, and pepper.
6. Spread the seasoned sweet potato cubes in a single layer on a baking sheet and roast in the preheated oven for about 20-25 minutes, or until they are tender and slightly caramelized.
7. Grill the marinated beef sirloin for about 4-5 minutes per side, or until it reaches your desired level of doneness (145°F / 63°C for medium-rare, 160°F / 71°C for medium). Let the steak rest for a few minutes before slicing.

Nutritional Values: Calories: 400 kcal | Fat: 20 g | Protein: 30 g | Carbs: 30 g | Net carbs: 22 g | Fiber: 8 g | Cholesterol: 85 mg | Sodium: 400 mg | Potassium: 1000 mg

Useful Tip: For a milder spice level, you can remove the seeds from the chipotle peppers before mincing them.

Fish Recipes

Lemon Herb Baked Salmon with Asparagus

Serving: 4 | Prep time: 15 minutes | Cook time: 20 minutes

Ingredients:

For the Lemon Herb Baked Salmon:

- 4 salmon fillets, skin-on
- 2 tbsp olive oil
- Zest of 1 lemon
- Juice of 1 lemon
- 2 cloves garlic, minced
- 1 tsp dried oregano
- Salt and pepper to taste

For the Asparagus:

- 1 bunch asparagus, ends trimmed
- 1 tbsp olive oil
- Salt and pepper to taste

Directions:

1. Preheat the oven to 400°F (200°C).
2. In a bowl, whisk together the olive oil, lemon zest, lemon juice, minced garlic, dried oregano, salt, and pepper to create the marinade.
3. Place the salmon fillets in a baking dish and pour the marinade over them. Make sure the fillets are coated with the marinade.
4. Arrange the trimmed asparagus around the salmon fillets in the baking dish. Drizzle the asparagus with olive oil and season with salt and pepper.
5. Bake the salmon and asparagus in the preheated oven for about 15-20 minutes, or until the salmon is cooked through and flakes easily with a fork.
6. Remove from the oven and serve the lemon herb baked salmon with the roasted asparagus on the side.

Nutritional Values: Calories: 350 kcal | Fat: 18 g | Protein: 30 g | Carbs: 15 g | Net carbs: 10 g | Fiber: 5 g | Cholesterol: 80 mg | Sodium: 350 mg | Potassium: 900 mg

Useful Tip: To prevent the salmon skin from sticking to the baking dish, you can place the fillets on parchment paper before adding the marinade.

Spicy Grilled Tilapia with Mango Salsa

Serving: 4 | Prep time: 15 minutes | Cook time: 10 minutes

Ingredients:

- 4 tilapia fillets
- 2 tbsp olive oil
- 1 tsp paprika
- 1/2 tsp cayenne pepper
- 1/2 tsp garlic powder
- Salt and pepper to taste

For Mango Salsa:

- 1 ripe mango, diced
- 1/4 red onion, finely chopped
- 1 small jalapeño, seeds removed and finely chopped
- 2 tbsp fresh cilantro, chopped
- 1 tbsp lime juice
- Salt to taste

Directions:

1. Preheat the grill to medium-high heat (about 375°F / 190°C).
2. In a small bowl, mix together the olive oil, paprika, cayenne pepper, garlic powder, salt, and pepper to create the marinade.
3. Rub the marinade onto both sides of the tilapia fillets.
4. Place the marinated fillets on the grill and cook for about 4-5 minutes on each side or until the fish flakes easily with a fork.
5. While the fish is grilling, prepare the mango salsa by combining the diced mango, red onion, jalapeño, cilantro, lime juice, and a pinch of salt in a bowl. Mix well.
6. Once the tilapia fillets are cooked, remove them from the grill.
7. Serve the grilled tilapia with a generous spoonful of mango salsa on top.

Useful Tip: You can adjust the level of spiciness by increasing or decreasing the amount of cayenne pepper in the marinade and adjusting the amount of jalapeño in the salsa according to your preference.

Nutritional Values: Calories: 245 kcal | Fat: 10 g | Protein: 33 g | Carbs: 10 g | Net carbs: 8 g | Fiber: 2 g | Cholesterol: 85 mg | Sodium: 80 mg | Potassium: 610 mg

Garlic Butter Cod with Roasted Brussels Sprouts

Serving: 4 | Prep time: 15 minutes | Cook time: 25 minutes

Ingredients:

- 4 cod fillets (5 oz / 140 g each)
- 2 tbsp unsalted butter, melted
- 3 cloves garlic, minced

- 1 tbsp fresh parsley, chopped
- Salt and pepper to taste

For Roasted Brussels Sprouts:

- 1 lb (450 g) Brussels sprouts, trimmed and halved
- 2 tbsp olive oil

- 1/2 tsp garlic powder
- Salt and pepper to taste

Directions:

1. Preheat the oven to 400°F (200°C).
2. Place the halved Brussels sprouts on a baking sheet, drizzle with olive oil, sprinkle with garlic powder, salt, and pepper, then toss to coat.
3. Roast the Brussels sprouts in the preheated oven for about 20-25 minutes or until they are golden brown and tender, stirring halfway through.
4. While the Brussels sprouts are roasting, prepare the garlic butter mixture for the cod by combining melted butter, minced garlic, chopped parsley, salt, and pepper in a bowl.
5. Season both sides of the cod fillets with salt and pepper.
6. Heat a skillet over medium-high heat and add a drizzle of olive oil.
7. Place the cod fillets in the skillet and cook for about 3-4 minutes on each side, or until they are cooked through and easily flake with a fork.
8. Pour the prepared garlic butter mixture over the cooked cod fillets in the skillet, allowing it to melt and coat the fish.
9. Serve the garlic butter cod fillets alongside the roasted Brussels sprouts.

Useful Tip: To achieve a nice golden-brown sear on the cod fillets, make sure the skillet is hot before adding the fish.

Nutritional Values: Calories: 275 kcal | Fat: 14 g | Protein: 30 g | Carbs: 12 g | Net carbs: 8 g | Fiber: 4 g | Cholesterol: 70 mg | Sodium: 210 mg | Potassium: 860 mg

Teriyaki Glazed Mahi-Mahi with Cauliflower Rice

Serving: 4 | Prep time: 15 minutes | Cook time: 20 minutes

Ingredients:

- 4 mahi-mahi fillets (6 oz / 170 g each)
- 4 tbsp low-sodium soy sauce
- 2 tbsp water
- 2 tbsp honey
- 1 tbsp rice vinegar
- 1 tsp ginger, minced
- 2 cloves garlic, minced

- 1 tbsp olive oil
- 1 medium head cauliflower, riced
- 1 carrot, finely chopped
- 3 oz (80 g) peas (fresh or frozen)
- 2 green onions, sliced
- Sesame seeds for garnish
- Salt and pepper to taste

Directions:

1. In a bowl, whisk together soy sauce, water, honey, rice vinegar, minced ginger, and minced garlic to create the teriyaki sauce.
2. Season the mahi-mahi fillets with a pinch of salt and pepper on both sides.
3. Heat olive oil in a skillet over medium-high heat.
4. Place the mahi-mahi fillets in the skillet and cook for about 3-4 minutes on each side, or until they are cooked through and have a nice sear.
5. Pour the teriyaki sauce over the cooked fillets in the skillet and let it simmer for an additional 1-2 minutes, allowing the sauce to glaze the fish.
6. While the fish is cooking, make the cauliflower rice by grating the cauliflower florets using a box grater or pulsing in a food processor until rice-like in texture.
7. In a separate skillet, heat a small amount of olive oil over medium heat.
8. Add the chopped carrot and peas, and sauté for about 3-4 minutes until the vegetables are tender.
9. Stir in the cauliflower rice and cook for another 3-4 minutes, stirring occasionally.
10. Season the cauliflower rice with salt and pepper to taste.
11. Serve the teriyaki glazed mahi-mahi over a bed of cauliflower rice, garnished with sliced green onions and sesame seeds.

Useful Tip: To achieve a beautiful glaze on the fish, make sure to brush the fillets with the teriyaki sauce as they cook.

Nutritional Values: Calories: 310 kcal | Fat: 8 g | Protein: 38 g | Carbs: 22 g | Net carbs: 16 g | Fiber: 6 g | Cholesterol: 120 mg | Sodium: 720 mg | Potassium: 1200 mg

Mediterranean-Style Grilled Sea Bass with Zucchini Noodles

Serving: 4 | Prep time: 20 minutes | Cook time: 15 minutes

Ingredients:

- 4 sea bass fillets (5 oz / 140 g each)
- 2 oz (60 ml) olive oil
- 2 cloves garlic, minced
- 1 tsp dried oregano
- 1 tsp dried thyme
- Zest and juice of 1 lemon
- Salt and pepper to taste

For Zucchini Noodles:

- 4 medium zucchinis (32 oz / 900 g), spiralized into noodles
- 2 tbsp olive oil
- 6 oz (170 g), cherry tomatoes , halved
- 1.75 oz (50 g) Kalamata olives, pitted and halved
- 2 tbsp fresh basil, chopped
- 1.75 oz (50 g) crumbled feta cheese
- Salt and pepper to taste

Directions:

1. Preheat the grill to medium-high heat.
2. In a bowl, whisk together olive oil, minced garlic, dried oregano, dried thyme, lemon zest, lemon juice, salt, and pepper to create the marinade.
3. Place the sea bass fillets in a shallow dish and pour the marinade over them. Let them marinate for about 10 minutes.
4. While the sea bass is marinating, heat 2 tablespoons of olive oil in a large skillet over medium heat.
5. Add the cherry tomatoes and sauté for about 3-4 minutes until they start to soften.
6. Stir in the spiralized zucchini noodles and cook for an additional 2-3 minutes, until the noodles are just tender.
7. Add the Kalamata olives and chopped basil to the skillet, and season with salt and pepper to taste.
8. Remove the sea bass fillets from the marinade and grill them for about 4-5 minutes on each side, or until they are cooked through and have nice grill marks.
9. Plate the grilled sea bass on a bed of zucchini noodles and top with crumbled feta cheese.

Useful Tip: To prevent the zucchini noodles from becoming too watery, avoid overcooking them - they should be cooked until just tender.

Nutritional Values: Calories: 320 kcal | Fat: 20 g | Protein: 28 g | Carbs: 12 g | Net carbs: 8 g | Fiber: 4 g | Cholesterol: 80 mg | Sodium: 580 mg | Potassium: 800 mg

Blackened Red Snapper Tacos with Avocado Crema

Serving: 4 | Prep time: 15 minutes | Cook time: 10 minutes

Ingredients:

- 4 red snapper fillets (5 oz / 140 g each)
- 1 tbsp paprika
- 1 tsp dried oregano
- 1 tsp garlic powder
- 1/2 tsp cayenne pepper
- 1/2 tsp onion powder
- 1/2 tsp salt
- 1/4 tsp black pepper
- 2 tbsp olive oil
- 8 small whole wheat or corn tortillas
- 2.5 oz (70 g) shredded lettuce
- 8 oz (225 g) diced tomatoes
- 2.5 oz (70 g) diced red onion
- 0.25 oz (7 g) chopped fresh cilantro

For Avocado Crema:

- 1 ripe avocado
- 2 oz (60 g) Greek yogurt
- 1 tbsp lime juice
- Salt to taste

Directions:

1. In a small bowl, mix together paprika, dried oregano, garlic powder, cayenne pepper, onion powder, salt, and black pepper to create the blackened seasoning.
2. Pat dry the red snapper fillets with paper towels, then rub both sides of each fillet with the blackened seasoning mixture.
3. Heat olive oil in a skillet over medium-high heat.
4. Place the red snapper fillets in the skillet and cook for about 3-4 minutes on each side, or until the fish is opaque and flakes easily.
5. While the fish is cooking, prepare the avocado crema by mashing the ripe avocado in a bowl and mixing it with Greek yogurt, lime juice, and a pinch of salt until smooth.
6. Warm the tortillas in a dry skillet or microwave.
7. To assemble the tacos, spread a spoonful of avocado crema onto each tortilla.
8. Top with shredded lettuce, diced tomatoes, red onion, and chopped cilantro.
9. Once the red snapper fillets are cooked, flake them with a fork and distribute the fish evenly among the tacos.

Useful Tip: To balance the heat of the blackened seasoning, the coolness of the avocado crema provides a delightful contrast.

Nutritional Values: Calories: 320 kcal | Fat: 12 g | Protein: 28 g | Carbs: 28 g | Net carbs: 24 g | Fiber: 4 g | Cholesterol: 60 mg | Sodium: 620 mg | Potassium: 700 mg

Sesame Crusted Tuna Steaks with Cucumber Salad

Serving: 4 | Prep time: 15 minutes | Cook time: 8 minutes

Ingredients:

- 4 tuna steaks (5 oz / 140 g each)
- 2 tbsp sesame seeds
- 1 tbsp black sesame seeds
- 1 tsp grated ginger

- 2 tbsp soy sauce
- 1 tbsp sesame oil
- 1 tbsp olive oil
- Salt and pepper to taste

For Cucumber Salad:

- 2 cucumbers, thinly sliced
- 1/4 red onion, thinly sliced
- 2 tbsp rice vinegar

- 1 tsp honey
- 1 tsp toasted sesame seeds
- Fresh cilantro leaves for garnish

Directions:

1. Preheat a non-stick skillet over medium-high heat.
2. In a shallow dish, combine the sesame seeds and black sesame seeds.
3. Rub both sides of the tuna steaks with grated ginger and drizzle with soy sauce.
4. Press the tuna steaks into the sesame seed mixture to coat them thoroughly.
5. In the preheated skillet, heat sesame oil and olive oil.
6. Place the coated tuna steaks in the skillet and cook for about 2-3 minutes on each side for medium-rare, or longer if desired.
7. While the tuna is cooking, prepare the cucumber salad by combining sliced cucumbers and red onion in a bowl.
8. In a separate bowl, whisk together rice vinegar, honey, and toasted sesame seeds to create the dressing.
9. Toss the cucumber and onion mixture with the dressing until well coated.
10. Plate the sesame crusted tuna steaks and serve them alongside the cucumber salad.

Useful Tip: To maintain the sesame crust's crunchiness, don't press too hard while searing the tuna.

Nutritional Values: Calories: 280 kcal | Fat: 13 g | Protein: 33 g | Carbs: 10 g | Net carbs: 7 g | Fiber: 3 g | Cholesterol: 55 mg | Sodium: 540 mg | Potassium: 850 mg

Herb-Marinated Grilled Trout with Lemon-Dill Sauce

Serving: 4 | Prep time: 20 minutes | Cook time: 10 minutes

Ingredients:

- 4 trout fillets (6 oz / 170 g each), skin on
- 2 tbsp olive oil
- 2 tbsp fresh parsley, chopped
- 1 tbsp fresh dill, chopped

- 1 tsp fresh thyme leaves
- 2 cloves garlic, minced
- Zest and juice of 1 lemon
- Salt and pepper to taste

For Lemon-Dill Sauce:

- 4 oz (120 g) Greek yogurt
- 1 tbsp fresh dill, chopped

- 1 tbsp lemon juice
- Salt to taste

Directions:

1. In a bowl, whisk together olive oil, chopped parsley, chopped dill, thyme leaves, minced garlic, lemon zest, lemon juice, salt, and pepper to create the marinade.
2. Place the trout fillets in a shallow dish and pour the marinade over them. Let them marinate for about 15 minutes.
3. Preheat the grill to medium-high heat.
4. Gently shake off excess marinade from the fillets and place them on the grill, skin side down.
5. Grill the trout fillets for about 3-4 minutes on each side, or until the fish flakes easily and the skin is crispy.
6. While the trout is grilling, prepare the lemon-dill sauce by mixing together Greek yogurt, chopped dill, lemon juice, and a pinch of salt in a bowl.
7. Once the trout is cooked, remove it from the grill and plate it.
8. Drizzle each fillet with the lemon-dill sauce.

Nutritional Values: Calories: 290 kcal | Fat: 15 g | Protein: 32 g | Carbs: 6 g | Net carbs: 4 g | Fiber: 2 g | Cholesterol: 80 mg | Sodium: 190 mg | Potassium: 620 mg

Useful Tip: To prevent sticking, ensure the grill grates are well-oiled before placing the trout fillets on them.

Coconut Lime Grilled Halibut with Broccoli and Quinoa

Serving: 4 | Prep time: 20 minutes | Cook time: 15 minutes

Ingredients:

- 4 halibut fillets (6 oz / 170 g each)
- 4 oz (120 ml) coconut milk
- Zest and juice of 2 limes
- 2 tbsp fresh cilantro, chopped

- 2 cloves garlic, minced
- 1 tsp ginger, minced
- Salt and pepper to taste

For Broccoli and Quinoa:

- 6 oz (170 g) broccoli florets
- 6 oz (170 g) quinoa , rinsed and drained
- 16 oz (480 ml) water

- 1 tbsp olive oil
- Salt to taste

Directions:

1. In a bowl, whisk together coconut milk, lime zest, lime juice, chopped cilantro, minced garlic, minced ginger, salt, and pepper to create the marinade.
2. Place the halibut fillets in a shallow dish and pour the marinade over them. Let them marinate for about 15 minutes.
3. Preheat the grill to medium-high heat.
4. In a medium saucepan, bring 2 cups of water to a boil. Add the rinsed quinoa, reduce the heat to low, cover, and let it simmer for about 15 minutes or until the quinoa is cooked and the water is absorbed.
5. While the quinoa is cooking, toss the broccoli florets with olive oil and a pinch of salt.
6. Place the marinated halibut fillets on the grill and cook for about 3-4 minutes on each side, or until the fish is cooked through and has nice grill marks.
7. During the last few minutes of grilling, add the broccoli florets to the grill and cook until they are tender and slightly charred.
8. Plate the grilled halibut fillets over a bed of cooked quinoa and grilled broccoli.

Nutritional Values: Calories: 350 kcal | Fat: 10 g | Protein: 30 g | Carbs: 35 g | Net carbs: 28 g | Fiber: 7 g | Cholesterol: 40 mg | Sodium: 280 mg | Potassium: 940 mg

Useful Tip: To prevent the halibut from sticking to the grill, make sure the grates are well-oiled and the fillets have a thin layer of marinade on them.

Pesto-Stuffed Whole Branzino with Roasted Carrots

Serving: 4 | Prep time: 25 minutes | Cook time: 25 minutes

Ingredients:

- 2 whole branzino fish (about 1 lb / 450 g each), cleaned and scaled
- 2 oz (60 g) prepared pesto
- Zest and juice of 1 lemon

- 2 cloves garlic, minced
- 1 oz (5 g) fresh basil leaves, chopped
- Salt and pepper to taste

For Roasted Carrots:

- 1 lb (450 g) baby carrots, washed and trimmed
- 2 tbsp olive oil

- 1 tsp dried thyme
- Salt and pepper to taste

Directions:

1. Preheat the oven to 400°F (200°C).
2. In a bowl, mix together prepared pesto, lemon zest, lemon juice, minced garlic, chopped basil, salt, and pepper to create the stuffing.
3. Make diagonal cuts on both sides of each branzino, creating small pockets for the stuffing.
4. Stuff each branzino with the prepared pesto mixture, distributing it evenly between the cuts.
5. Place the stuffed branzino on a baking sheet lined with parchment paper.
6. In a separate bowl, toss baby carrots with olive oil, dried thyme, salt, and pepper.
7. Arrange the seasoned carrots around the stuffed branzino on the baking sheet.
8. Roast in the preheated oven for about 20-25 minutes, or until the fish flakes easily and the carrots are tender.
9. While the branzino is roasting, the stuffing will infuse the fish with flavor and keep it moist.

Nutritional Values: Calories: 300 kcal | Fat: 14 g | Protein: 28 g | Carbs: 16 g | Net carbs: 12 g | Fiber: 4 g | Cholesterol: 60 mg | Sodium: 400 mg | Potassium: 900 mg

Useful Tip: Score the skin of the branzino to ensure even cooking and better flavor absorption.

Seafood Recipes

Creamy Garlic Lemon Butter Shrimp with Zucchini Noodles

Serving: 4 | Prep time: 15 minutes | Cook time: 10 minutes

Ingredients:

- 1 lb (450 g) large shrimp, peeled and deveined
- 2 tbsp unsalted butter
- 4 cloves garlic, minced
- Zest and juice of 1 lemon
- 4 oz (120 ml) heavy cream
- 1oz (28 g) grated Parmesan cheese
- 2 medium zucchinis (16 oz / 450 g), spiralized into noodles
- 2 tbsp fresh parsley, chopped
- Salt and pepper to taste

Directions:

1. In a skillet over medium-high heat, melt the butter.
2. Add the minced garlic and cook for about 1 minute until fragrant.
3. Add the shrimp to the skillet and cook for 2-3 minutes on each side, until they turn pink and opaque.
4. Remove the shrimp from the skillet and set them aside.
5. In the same skillet, pour in the heavy cream and bring it to a gentle simmer.
6. Stir in the grated Parmesan cheese until it's fully melted into the cream.
7. Add the lemon zest and lemon juice to the creamy sauce, and season with salt and pepper to taste.
8. Return the cooked shrimp to the skillet and toss them in the creamy sauce to coat.
9. Add the spiralized zucchini noodles to the skillet and cook for about 2-3 minutes until they are just tender.
10. Garnish the dish with chopped fresh parsley.

Nutritional Values: Calories: 350 kcal | Fat: 22 g | Protein: 30 g | Carbs: 10 g | Net carbs: 6 g | Fiber: 4 g | Cholesterol: 270 mg | Sodium: 450 mg | Potassium: 600 mg

Useful Tip: If you prefer a thicker sauce, allow it to simmer a bit longer before adding the shrimp back in.

Spicy Coconut Curry Scallops with Cauliflower Rice

Serving: 4 | Prep time: 20 minutes | Cook time: 15 minutes

Ingredients:

- 1 lb (450 g) scallops
- 2 oz (28 g) coconut oil
- 1 onion, finely chopped
- 2 cloves garlic, minced
- 1 tbsp ginger, minced
- 0.5 oz (14 g) red curry paste
- 13.5 oz (400 ml) can of coconut milk
- 6 oz (170 g) bell peppers, thinly sliced
- 4 oz (115 g) snap peas, ends trimmed
- 1 tbsp fish sauce
- 1 tbsp lime juice
- 1 tsp honey
- Fresh cilantro leaves for garnish

For Cauliflower Rice:

- 16 oz (450 g) medium cauliflower, riced
- 0.5 oz (14 g) coconut oil
- Salt and pepper to taste

Directions:

1. In a large skillet, heat coconut oil over medium heat.
2. Add chopped onion and sauté for about 2-3 minutes until softened.
3. Stir in minced garlic and ginger, and cook for another 1 minute.
4. Add red curry paste to the skillet and cook for 1-2 minutes to release its flavors.
5. Pour in the coconut milk and bring to a gentle simmer.
6. Add sliced bell peppers and snap peas to the skillet, and cook for 3-4 minutes until slightly tender.
7. Stir in fish sauce, lime juice, and honey to the curry sauce.
8. In a separate skillet, heat coconut oil over medium heat.
9. Add riced cauliflower and cook for about 5-6 minutes until it's tender and slightly golden.
10. While the cauliflower rice is cooking, season the scallops with salt and pepper.
11. Heat a separate skillet over high heat and sear the scallops for about 1-2 minutes on each side until they're nicely browned and cooked through.
12. Plate the cauliflower rice, top with the spicy coconut curry sauce, and place the seared scallops on top.
13. Garnish with fresh cilantro leaves.

Nutritional Values: Calories: 350 kcal | Fat: 18 g | Protein: 25 g | Carbs: 28 g | Net carbs: 20 g | Fiber: 8 g | Cholesterol: 40 mg | Sodium: 700 mg | Potassium: 1200 mg

Useful Tip: For perfectly seared scallops, make sure the skillet is hot before adding them.

Grilled Lemon Herb Prawns with Roasted Brussels Sprouts

Serving: 4 | Prep time: 20 minutes | Cook time: 15 minutes

Ingredients:

- 1 lb (450 g) large prawns, peeled and deveined
- 2 tbsp olive oil
- Zest and juice of 1 lemon
- 2 cloves garlic, minced

- 2 tbsp fresh parsley, chopped
- 1 tsp dried oregano
- Salt and pepper to taste

For Roasted Brussels Sprouts:

- 1 lb (450 g) Brussels sprouts, trimmed and halved
- 2 tbsp olive oil
- 1/2 tsp garlic powder

- Salt and pepper to taste
- Skewers

Directions:

1. Preheat the grill to medium-high heat.
2. In a bowl, whisk together olive oil, lemon zest, lemon juice, minced garlic, chopped parsley, dried oregano, salt, and pepper.
3. Add the prawns to the bowl and toss to coat them in the marinade. Let them marinate for about 10 minutes.
4. In another bowl, toss halved Brussels sprouts with olive oil, garlic powder, salt, and pepper.
5. Thread the marinated prawns onto skewers.
6. Grill the prawn skewers for about 2-3 minutes on each side until they are pink and cooked through.
7. While the prawns are grilling, preheat the oven to 400°F (200°C) for roasting the Brussels sprouts.
8. Spread the seasoned Brussels sprouts on a baking sheet in a single layer and roast them in the preheated oven for about 12-15 minutes until they are crispy and golden.
9. Serve the grilled lemon herb prawns alongside the roasted Brussels sprouts.

Nutritional Values: Calories: 300 kcal | Fat: 15 g | Protein: 25 g | Carbs: 20 g | Net carbs: 15 g | Fiber: 5 g | Cholesterol: 180 mg | Sodium: 450 mg | Potassium: 900 mg

Useful Tip: Soak wooden skewers in water for 30 minutes before grilling to prevent them from burning.

Cajun Spiced Grilled Shrimp Tacos with Avocado Salsa

Serving: 4 | Prep time: 20 minutes | Cook time: 10 minutes

Ingredients:

- 1 lb (450 g) large shrimp, peeled and deveined
- 1 tbsp olive oil

- 1 tbsp Cajun seasoning
- 8 small corn tortillas

For Avocado Salsa:

- 2 ripe avocados, diced
- 1 small red onion, finely chopped
- 1 small tomato, diced
- 1 jalapeño, seeded and finely chopped

- Juice of 1 lime
- 2 tbsp fresh cilantro, chopped
- Salt and pepper to taste

Directions:

1. In a bowl, toss the shrimp with olive oil and Cajun seasoning until well coated.
2. Preheat the grill to medium-high heat.
3. Thread the seasoned shrimp onto skewers.
4. Grill the shrimp skewers for about 2-3 minutes on each side until they are pink and cooked through.
5. While the shrimp are grilling, prepare the avocado salsa by combining diced avocados, chopped red onion, diced tomato, chopped jalapeño, lime juice, chopped cilantro, salt, and pepper in a bowl. Gently mix to combine.
6. Warm the corn tortillas on the grill for about 20-30 seconds on each side.
7. To assemble the tacos, place a few grilled shrimp on each tortilla and top with a generous spoonful of avocado salsa.

Nutritional Values: Calories: 280 kcal | Fat: 10 g | Protein: 18 g | Carbs: 32 g | Net carbs: 25 g | Fiber: 7 g | Cholesterol: 150 mg | Sodium: 300 mg | Potassium: 700 mg

Useful Tip: If using wooden skewers, soak them in water for about 30 minutes before grilling to prevent them from burning.

Thai Coconut Curry Mussels with Zucchini Noodles

Serving: 4 | Prep time: 15 minutes | Cook time: 15 minutes

Ingredients:

- 2 lbs (900 g) fresh mussels, cleaned and debearded
- 2 tbsp coconut oil
- 1 onion, thinly sliced
- 2 cloves garlic, minced
- 1 tbsp ginger, minced
- 2 tbsp Thai red curry paste
- 1 can (13.5 oz / 400 ml) coconut milk
- 6 oz (170 g) cherry tomatoes, halved
- 2 medium zucchinis (16 oz / 450 g), spiralized into noodles
- Juice of 1 lime
- Fresh cilantro leaves for garnish
- Salt and pepper to taste

Directions:

1. In a large pot, heat coconut oil over medium heat.
2. Add sliced onion and sauté for about 2-3 minutes until softened.
3. Stir in minced garlic and ginger, and cook for another 1 minute.
4. Add Thai red curry paste to the pot and cook for 1-2 minutes to release its flavors.
5. Pour in the coconut milk and bring to a gentle simmer.
6. Add cleaned mussels and halved cherry tomatoes to the pot. Cover with a lid and cook for 5-7 minutes, shaking the pot occasionally, until the mussels open.
7. While the mussels are cooking, heat a separate skillet over medium heat.
8. Add spiralized zucchini noodles to the skillet and cook for about 2-3 minutes until they are just tender.
9. Once the mussels are cooked and open, discard any that remain closed.
10. Stir in the juice of 1 lime to the mussels and adjust the seasoning with salt and pepper.
11. Plate the zucchini noodles, top with the Thai coconut curry mussels, and garnish with fresh cilantro leaves.

Nutritional Values: Calories: 350 kcal | Fat: 20 g | Protein: 25 g | Carbs: 20 g | Net carbs: 12 g | Fiber: 8 g | Cholesterol: 70 mg | Sodium: 550 mg | Potassium: 1200 mg

Useful Tip: Make sure to clean and debeard the mussels thoroughly before cooking.

Herb-Crusted Baked Lobster Tail with Garlic Mashed Cauliflower

Serving: 4 | Prep time: 20 minutes | Cook time: 25 minutes

Ingredients:

- 4 lobster tails (about 8 oz / 225 g each)
- 2 oz (56 g) butter, melted
- 4 oz (115 g) almond flour
- 0.25 oz (7 g) fresh parsley, finely chopped
- 1 tsp dried thyme
- 1 tsp dried rosemary
- Salt and pepper to taste

For Garlic Mashed Cauliflower:

- 1 head cauliflower, cut into florets (about 2 lbs / 900 g)
- 4 cloves garlic, minced
- 2 oz (56 g) cream cheese
- 2 oz (56 g) butter
- Salt and pepper to taste

Directions:

1. Preheat the oven to 400°F (200°C).
2. In a bowl, combine almond flour, chopped parsley, dried thyme, dried rosemary, salt, and pepper to create the herb crust mixture.
3. Carefully split the top of each lobster tail shell lengthwise, exposing the meat.
4. Brush the lobster meat with melted butter and press the herb crust mixture onto the buttered lobster meat.
5. Place the lobster tails on a baking sheet lined with parchment paper and bake in the preheated oven for about 15-20 minutes until the lobster meat is opaque and cooked through.
6. While the lobster tails are baking, steam the cauliflower florets until they are tender.
7. In a pot, melt the butter and sauté the minced garlic until fragrant.
8. Add the steamed cauliflower to the pot and use a potato masher to mash it.
9. Stir in cream cheese until the cauliflower is creamy and smooth. Season with salt and pepper.
10. Serve the herb-crusted baked lobster tails alongside the garlic mashed cauliflower.

Nutritional Values: Calories: 350 kcal | Fat: 25 g | Protein: 20 g | Carbs: 12 g | Net carbs: 8 g | Fiber: 4 g | Cholesterol: 150 mg | Sodium: 600 mg | Potassium: 700 mg

Useful Tip: To split the lobster tail shell, use kitchen shears to carefully cut along the center line of the shell.

Lemon Dill Garlic Butter Crab Cakes with Asparagus Spears

Serving: 4 | Prep time: 25 minutes | Cook time: 15 minutes

Ingredients:

- 1 lb (450 g) lump crab meat
- 2 tbsp almond flour
- 1 egg
- 2 cloves garlic, minced

- Zest and juice of 1 lemon
- 2 tbsp fresh dill, chopped
- 2 tbsp butter, melted
- Salt and pepper to taste

For Asparagus Spears:

- 1 bunch asparagus spears, trimmed
- 2 tbsp olive oil

- Salt and pepper to taste

Directions:

1. Preheat the oven to 375°F (190°C).
2. In a bowl, combine lump crab meat, almond flour, minced garlic, lemon zest, lemon juice, chopped dill, melted butter, salt, and pepper.
3. Gently fold in the beaten egg until the mixture is well combined.
4. Shape the crab mixture into 8 equal-sized patties.
5. Place the crab cakes on a baking sheet lined with parchment paper and bake in the preheated oven for about 12-15 minutes until they are golden brown and cooked through.
6. While the crab cakes are baking, toss trimmed asparagus spears with olive oil, salt, and pepper.
7. Roast the asparagus in the preheated oven for about 8-10 minutes until they are tender.
8. Serve the lemon dill garlic butter crab cakes alongside the roasted asparagus spears.

Nutritional Values: Calories: 280 kcal | Fat: 15 g | Protein: 20 g | Carbs: 8 g | Net carbs: 5 g | Fiber: 3 g | Cholesterol: 150 mg | Sodium: 600 mg | Potassium: 700 mg

Useful Tip: Be gentle when shaping the crab cakes to maintain the lump texture of the crab meat.

Mediterranean-Style Grilled Squid with Tomato Olive Relish

Serving: 4 | Prep time: 20 minutes | Cook time: 8 minutes

Ingredients:

- 1 lb (450 g) cleaned squid tubes
- 2 tbsp olive oil
- Juice of 1 lemon

- 2 cloves garlic, minced
- 1 tsp dried oregano
- Salt and pepper to taste

For Tomato Olive Relish:

- 5 oz (140 g) cherry tomatoes, halved
- 1.5 oz (42 g) Kalamata olives, pitted and chopped
- 2 tbsp red onion, finely chopped
- 2 tbsp fresh parsley, chopped

- 1 tbsp olive oil
- Juice of 1 lemon
- Salt and pepper to taste
- Skewers

Directions:

1. Preheat the grill to medium-high heat.
2. In a bowl, whisk together olive oil, lemon juice, minced garlic, dried oregano, salt, and pepper.
3. Pat the cleaned squid tubes dry and score them in a crisscross pattern on one side.
4. Toss the squid tubes in the marinade, making sure they are well coated. Let them marinate for about 10 minutes.
5. While the squid is marinating, prepare the tomato olive relish by combining halved cherry tomatoes, chopped olives, finely chopped red onion, chopped parsley, olive oil, lemon juice, salt, and pepper in a bowl.
6. Thread the marinated squid tubes onto skewers.
7. Grill the squid skewers for about 2-3 minutes on each side until they are cooked and have grill marks.
8. Serve the grilled squid skewers with the tomato olive relish on top.

Nutritional Values: Calories: 220 kcal | Fat: 12 g | Protein: 18 g | Carbs: 10 g | Net carbs: 6 g | Fiber: 4 g | Cholesterol: 250 mg | Sodium: 600 mg | Potassium: 600 mg

Useful Tip: To prevent squid from becoming tough, avoid overcooking—grill them just until they turn opaque and firm

Teriyaki Glazed Grilled Octopus Skewers with Stir-Fried Bok Choy

Serving: 4 | Prep time: 20 minutes | Cook time: 10 minutes

Ingredients:

- 1 lb (450 g) octopus tentacles, cleaned and cooked
- 2 tbsp soy sauce
- 2 tbsp mirin
- 1 tbsp sake
- 1 tbsp honey
- 1 tsp sesame oil
- 2 cloves garlic, minced
- 1 tsp ginger, minced
- 2 baby bok choy, halved and cleaned
- 1 tbsp olive oil
- 2 cloves garlic, minced
- 1 tsp ginger, minced
- 2 baby bok choy, halved and cleaned

Directions:

1. In a bowl, whisk together soy sauce, mirin, sake, honey, sesame oil, minced garlic, and minced ginger to make the teriyaki marinade.
2. Cut the cooked octopus tentacles into bite-sized pieces and marinate them in the teriyaki sauce for about 10 minutes.
3. Preheat the grill to medium-high heat.
4. Thread the marinated octopus pieces onto skewers.
5. Grill the octopus skewers for about 2-3 minutes on each side, basting them with the remaining teriyaki marinade.
6. While the octopus is grilling, heat olive oil in a pan over medium heat for the stir-fried bok choy.
7. Stir-fry the halved bok choy for 2-3 minutes until they are slightly tender and bright green.
8. Serve the teriyaki glazed octopus skewers on a bed of stir-fried bok choy.

Nutritional Values: Calories: 250 kcal | Fat: 10 g | Protein: 25 g | Carbs: 15 g | Net carbs: 12 g | Fiber: 3 g | Cholesterol: 120 mg | Sodium: 800 mg | Potassium: 700 mg

Useful Tip: Octopus can become rubbery if overcooked, so be sure to grill it just until it's heated through.

Citrus Herb Marinated Grilled Scallops with Lemon-Herb Quinoa

Serving: 4 | Prep time: 15 minutes | Cook time: 15 minutes

Ingredients:

- 1 lb (450 g) fresh scallops
- Zest and juice of 1 lemon
- Zest and juice of 1 orange
- 2 tbsp olive oil
- 2 cloves garlic, minced
- 1 lb (450 g) fresh scallops
- Zest and juice of 1 lemon
- Zest and juice of 1 orange
- 2 tbsp olive oil
- 2 cloves garlic, minced
- 2 tbsp fresh parsley, chopped
- 1 tsp fresh thyme leaves
- Salt and pepper to taste
- 6 oz (170 g) quinoa
- 16 oz (473 ml) vegetable broth
- 1 lemon, cut into wedges for serving

Directions:

1. In a bowl, whisk together the lemon zest, orange zest, lemon juice, orange juice, olive oil, minced garlic, chopped parsley, fresh thyme leaves, salt, and pepper to make the marinade.
2. Pat the scallops dry and place them in a resealable plastic bag. Pour the marinade over the scallops, seal the bag, and refrigerate for about 15-20 minutes.
3. While the scallops are marinating, rinse the quinoa under cold water and drain.
4. In a saucepan, combine the quinoa and vegetable broth. Bring to a boil, then reduce the heat to low, cover, and simmer for about 15 minutes, or until the quinoa is cooked and the liquid is absorbed. Fluff with a fork and set aside.
5. Preheat the grill to medium-high heat.
6. Thread the marinated scallops onto skewers.
7. Grill the scallop skewers for about 2-3 minutes on each side until they are opaque and cooked through.
8. Serve the grilled scallops over a bed of lemon-herb quinoa and garnish with lemon wedges.

Nutritional Values: Calories: 320 kcal | Fat: 8 g | Protein: 25 g | Carbs: 40 g | Net carbs: 35 g | Fiber: 5 g | Cholesterol: 40 mg | Sodium: 800 mg | Potassium: 600 mg

Useful Tip: To prevent sticking, make sure the grill grates are clean and well-oiled before placing the scallops on them.

Chapter 4. Salads

Mediterranean Chickpea Salad with Lemon Herb Dressing

Serving: 4 | Prep time: 15 minutes | Cook time: 0 minutes

Ingredients:

- 15 oz (425 g each) chickpeas, drained and rinsed
- 15 oz (150 g) cherry tomatoes, halved
- 1 cucumber, diced
- 1/2 red onion, finely chopped

- 2 oz (75 g) Kalamata olives, pitted and halved
- 4 oz (70 g) crumbled feta cheese
- 4 oz (30 g) chopped fresh parsley

For Lemon Herb Dressing:

- 3 tbsp olive oil
- Juice of 1 lemon
- 2 cloves garlic, minced

- 1 tsp dried oregano
- Salt and pepper to taste

Directions:

1. In a large bowl, combine the chickpeas, cherry tomatoes, cucumber, red onion, Kalamata olives, crumbled feta cheese, and chopped parsley.
2. In a small bowl, whisk together olive oil, lemon juice, minced garlic, dried oregano, salt, and pepper to make the dressing.
3. Pour the lemon herb dressing over the chickpea mixture and toss well to combine.
4. Let the salad sit for about 10-15 minutes to allow the flavors to meld.
5. Serve the Mediterranean chickpea salad as a refreshing and nutritious side dish.

Nutritional Values: Calories: 320 kcal | Fat: 14 g | Protein: 10 g | Carbs: 38 g | Net carbs: 30 g | Fiber: 8 g | Cholesterol: 15 mg | Sodium: 500 mg | Potassium: 600 mg

Useful Tip: For added protein, you can toss in some grilled chicken or cooked quinoa into the salad.

Thai-Inspired Quinoa Salad with Peanut Lime Dressing

Serving: 4 | Prep time: 15 minutes | Cook time: 15 minutes

Ingredients:

- 3.5 oz (100 g) quinoa, rinsed and drained
- 16 oz (475 ml) water
- 1 red bell pepper, diced
- 5.3 oz (150 g) edamame beans, cooked and shelled

- 1 carrot, julienned
- 1.1 oz (30 g) chopped fresh cilantro
- 1.1 oz (30 g) chopped fresh mint
- 1.1 oz (30 g) chopped roasted peanuts

For Peanut Lime Dressing:

- 3 tbsp peanut butter
- 2 tbsp lime juice
- 2 tbsp soy sauce
- 1 tbsp sesame oil

- 1 tbsp honey
- 1 tsp grated fresh ginger
- 1 clove garlic, minced
- Red pepper flakes to taste

Directions:

1. In a medium saucepan, combine quinoa and water. Bring to a boil, then reduce the heat to low, cover, and simmer for about 15 minutes or until the quinoa is cooked and the water is absorbed.
2. In a large bowl, combine cooked quinoa, diced red bell pepper, edamame beans , julienned carrot, chopped cilantro, chopped mint, and chopped roasted peanuts.
3. In a small bowl, whisk together peanut butter, lime juice, soy sauce, sesame oil, honey, grated ginger, minced garlic, and red pepper flakes to make the dressing.
4. Pour the peanut lime dressing over the quinoa mixture and toss well to coat.
5. Serve the Thai-inspired quinoa salad as a flavorful and nutritious meal.

Nutritional Values: Calories: 380 kcal | Fat: 17 g | Protein: 14 g | Carbs: 42 g | Net carbs: 30 g | Fiber: 12 g | Cholesterol: 0 mg | Sodium: 600 mg | Potassium: 720 mg

Useful Tip: For a protein boost, you can add grilled chicken or tofu to the salad.

Roasted Beet and Goat Cheese Salad with Citrus Vinaigrette

Serving: 4 | Prep time: 15 minutes | Cook time: 40 minutes

Ingredients:

- 14.1 oz (400 g) beets (mixed colors), peeled and cubed
- 1.8 oz (50 g) mixed greens (e.g., arugula, spinach, lettuce)
- 2.1 oz (60 g) goat cheese, crumbled
- 1.4 oz (40 g) walnuts, chopped and toasted

For Citrus Vinaigrette:

- 1.5 oz (42 ml) olive oil
- 1 oz (30 ml) orange juice
- 0.5 oz (15 ml) lemon juice
- 1 tsp honey
- 0.18 oz (5 g) Dijon mustard
- Salt and pepper to taste

Directions:

1. Preheat the oven to 400°F (200°C).
2. Toss the cubed beets with a drizzle of olive oil and spread them on a baking sheet. Roast in the preheated oven for about 30-40 minutes until tender and slightly caramelized.
3. In a bowl, whisk together olive oil, orange juice, lemon juice, honey, Dijon mustard, salt, and pepper to make the citrus vinaigrette.
4. In a large salad bowl, combine the roasted beets, mixed greens, crumbled goat cheese, and toasted walnuts.
5. Drizzle the citrus vinaigrette over the salad and toss gently to coat.
6. Serve the roasted beet and goat cheese salad as a vibrant and delicious meal.

Nutritional Values: Calories: 280 kcal | Fat: 20 g | Protein: 7 g | Carbs: 19 g | Net carbs: 14 g | Fiber: 5 g | Cholesterol: 15 mg | Sodium: 200 mg | Potassium: 570 mg

Useful Tip: To easily peel the beets, you can wrap them in aluminum foil and roast them whole before peeling and cubing.

Roasted Sweet Potato and Kale Salad with Tahini Drizzle

Serving: 4 | Prep time: 15 minutes | Cook time: 25 minutes

Ingredients:

- 17.6 oz (500 g) sweet potatoes, peeled and cubed
- 5.3 oz (150 g) kale, stems removed and leaves torn
- 1.8 oz (50 g) red onion, thinly sliced
- 1.4 oz (40 g) pumpkin seeds, toasted
- 1.5 oz (42 ml) olive oil

For Tahini Drizzle:

- 2 oz (60 ml) tahini
- 1 oz (30 ml) lemon juice
- 1 oz (30 ml) water
- 1 clove garlic, minced
- Salt and pepper to taste

Directions:

1. Preheat the oven to 400°F (200°C).
2. Toss the cubed sweet potatoes with a drizzle of olive oil, salt, and pepper. Spread them on a baking sheet and roast for about 20-25 minutes until tender and slightly caramelized.
3. In a large mixing bowl, massage the torn kale leaves with a drizzle of olive oil for a few minutes until they soften.
4. In a small bowl, whisk together tahini, lemon juice, water, minced garlic, salt, and pepper to make the tahini drizzle.
5. Assemble the salad by arranging the massaged kale, roasted sweet potatoes, sliced red onion, and toasted pumpkin seeds on a serving platter.
6. Drizzle the tahini dressing over the salad.
7. Serve the roasted sweet potato and kale salad with the creamy tahini drizzle for a satisfying and nutrient-rich meal.

Nutritional Values: Calories: 320 kcal | Fat: 20 g | Protein: 9 g | Carbs: 30 g | Net carbs: 20 g | Fiber: 10 g | Cholesterol: 0 mg | Sodium: 180 mg | Potassium: 860 mg

Useful Tip: Massaging the kale with a bit of olive oil helps to soften its texture and make it more palatable.

Strawberry Spinach Salad with Poppy Seed Dressing

Serving: 4 | Prep time: 15 minutes | Cook time: 0 minutes

Ingredients:

- 10.6 oz (300 g) fresh spinach leaves, washed and dried
- 7 oz (200 g) strawberries, hulled and sliced
- 2 oz (60 g) red onion, thinly sliced
- 2 oz (60 g) toasted almonds, chopped

For Poppy Seed Dressing:

- 1 oz (30 ml) olive oil
- 1 oz (30 ml) apple cider vinegar
- 0.5 oz (15 ml) honey
- 0.5 oz (15 ml) Dijon mustard
- 1 tsp poppy seeds
- Salt and pepper to taste

Directions:

1. In a large salad bowl, combine the fresh spinach leaves, sliced strawberries, and thinly sliced red onion.
2. In a small bowl, whisk together olive oil, apple cider vinegar, honey, Dijon mustard, poppy seeds, salt, and pepper to make the poppy seed dressing.
3. Drizzle the poppy seed dressing over the salad ingredients.
4. Toss the salad gently to coat the ingredients with the dressing.
5. Sprinkle the chopped toasted almonds over the top.
6. Serve the strawberry spinach salad with poppy seed dressing as a refreshing and nutrient-packed meal.

Nutritional Values: Calories: 250 kcal | Fat: 15 g | Protein: 6 g | Carbs: 26 g | Net carbs: 20 g | Fiber: 6 g | Cholesterol: 0 mg | Sodium: 180 mg | Potassium: 600 mg

Useful Tip: To toast almonds, simply place them in a dry skillet over medium heat for a few minutes until they become fragrant and slightly browned.

Greek Cucumber and Feta Salad with Oregano Vinaigrette

Serving: 4 | Prep time: 15 minutes | Cook time: 0 minutes

Ingredients:

- 10.6 oz (300 g) cucumbers, sliced
- 6.7 oz (190 g) cherry tomatoes, halved
- 4 oz (115 g) feta cheese, crumbled
- 2 oz (60 g) red onion, thinly sliced
- 2 oz (60 g) Kalamata olives, pitted and halved

For Oregano Vinaigrette:

- 1 oz (30 ml) extra virgin olive oil
- 1 oz (30 ml) red wine vinegar
- 1 tsp dried oregano
- Salt and pepper to taste

Directions:

1. In a large salad bowl, combine the sliced cucumbers, halved cherry tomatoes, crumbled feta cheese, thinly sliced red onion, and halved Kalamata olives.
2. In a small bowl, whisk together extra virgin olive oil, red wine vinegar, dried oregano, salt, and pepper to make the oregano vinaigrette.
3. Drizzle the oregano vinaigrette over the salad ingredients.
4. Gently toss the salad to coat the ingredients with the vinaigrette.
5. Serve the Greek cucumber and feta salad as a refreshing and flavorful side dish.

Nutritional Values: Calories: 220 kcal | Fat: 18 g | Protein: 6 g | Carbs: 9 g | Net carbs: 7 g | Fiber: 2 g | Cholesterol: 35 mg | Sodium: 520 mg | Potassium: 300 mg

Useful Tip: For a more intense flavor, allow the salad to marinate in the refrigerator for about 30 minutes before serving.

Apple Walnut Salad with Maple Dijon Dressing

Serving: 4 | Prep time: 15 minutes | Cook time: 0 minutes

Ingredients:

- 10.6 oz (300 g) mixed salad greens
- 2 apples, cored and thinly sliced
- 3.5 oz (100 g) walnuts, toasted and chopped
- 2 oz (60 g) red onion, thinly sliced

For Maple Dijon Dressing:

- 1 oz (30 ml) olive oil
- 1 oz (30 ml) apple cider vinegar
- 0.5 oz (15 ml) pure maple syrup
- 1 tsp Dijon mustard
- Salt and pepper to taste

Directions:

1. In a large salad bowl, combine the mixed salad greens, thinly sliced apples, chopped toasted walnuts, and thinly sliced red onion.
2. In a small bowl, whisk together olive oil, apple cider vinegar, pure maple syrup, Dijon mustard, salt, and pepper to make the maple Dijon dressing.
3. Drizzle the maple Dijon dressing over the salad ingredients.
4. Gently toss the salad to coat the ingredients with the dressing.
5. Serve the apple walnut salad as a delightful and nutritious dish.

Nutritional Values: Calories: 280 kcal | Fat: 20 g | Protein: 4 g | Carbs: 23 g | Net carbs: 18 g | Fiber: 5 g | Cholesterol: 0 mg | Sodium: 60 mg | Potassium: 320 mg

Useful Tip: To toast walnuts, spread them in a single layer on a baking sheet and roast in a preheated oven at 350°F (175°C) for about 5-7 minutes until fragrant and lightly golden.

Caprese Salad with Fresh Basil and Balsamic Glaze

Serving: 4 | Prep time: 10 minutes | Cook time: 0 minutes

Ingredients:

- 12 oz (340 g) fresh mozzarella cheese, sliced
- 2 large tomatoes, sliced
- 1 oz (30 g) fresh basil leaves

For Balsamic Glaze:

- 2 oz (60 ml) balsamic vinegar
- 1 tbsp honey
- Salt and pepper to taste

Directions:

1. Arrange the slices of fresh mozzarella cheese and tomato on a serving platter, alternating them.
2. Tuck fresh basil leaves between the slices of cheese and tomato.
3. In a small saucepan, combine balsamic vinegar and honey for the balsamic glaze.
4. Bring the mixture to a gentle simmer over low heat, stirring occasionally, until it reduces by half and becomes slightly thicker.
5. Remove the balsamic glaze from heat and let it cool slightly.
6. Drizzle the balsamic glaze over the caprese salad.
7. Season the salad with salt and pepper to taste.
8. Serve the caprese salad with fresh basil and balsamic glaze as a light and flavorful dish.

Nutritional Values: Calories: 220 kcal | Fat: 14 g | Protein: 14 g | Carbs: 12 g | Net carbs: 10 g | Fiber: 2 g | Cholesterol: 40 mg | Sodium: 350 mg | Potassium: 450 mg

Useful Tip: To easily chiffonade the basil leaves, stack the leaves on top of each other, roll them tightly, and then slice crosswise into thin ribbons.

Asian Sesame Chicken Salad with Ginger Soy Dressing

Serving: 4 | Prep time: 20 minutes | Cook time: 10 minutes

Ingredients:

- 1 lb (450 g) boneless, skinless chicken breast, cooked and sliced
- 6 oz (170 g) mixed salad greens
- 1 large carrot, julienned
- 1 red bell pepper, thinly sliced
- 2 green onions, sliced
- 2 oz (60 g) toasted sesame seeds
- 1 oz (30 g) sliced almonds, toasted

For Ginger Soy Dressing:

- 2 oz (60 ml) soy sauce
- 1 oz (30 ml) rice vinegar
- 1 oz (30 ml) sesame oil
- 1 tbsp fresh ginger, grated
- 1 clove garlic, minced
- 1 tsp honey

Directions:

1. In a large salad bowl, combine the mixed salad greens, julienned carrot, red bell pepper slices, and sliced green onions.
2. Top the salad with the cooked and sliced chicken breast.
3. In a small bowl, whisk together the soy sauce, rice vinegar, sesame oil, grated ginger, minced garlic, and honey to make the ginger soy dressing.
4. Drizzle the ginger soy dressing over the salad.
5. Sprinkle the toasted sesame seeds and sliced almonds on top.
6. Toss the salad gently to combine all the ingredients and coat them with the dressing.
7. Serve the Asian sesame chicken salad with ginger soy dressing as a satisfying and flavorful meal.

Nutritional Values: Calories: 350 kcal | Fat: 20 g | Protein: 28 g | Carbs: 15 g | Net carbs: 10 g | Fiber: 5 g | Cholesterol: 70 mg | Sodium: 750 mg | Potassium: 550 mg

Useful Tip: To toast sesame seeds and sliced almonds, spread them on a baking sheet and bake in a preheated oven at 350°F (175°C) for about 5-7 minutes, stirring occasionally, until they are golden and fragrant.

Roasted Vegetable Salad with Herbed Yogurt Dressing

Serving: 4 | Prep time: 15 minutes | Cook time: 25 minutes

Ingredients:

- 16 oz (450 g) mixed vegetables (such as bell peppers, zucchini, and carrots), cut into bite-sized pieces
- 2 oz (60 ml) olive oil
- Salt and pepper to taste
- 6 oz (170 g) mixed salad greens
- 2 oz (60 g) cherry tomatoes, halved
- 1 oz (30 g) red onion, thinly sliced
- 2 oz (60 g) feta cheese, crumbled

For Herbed Yogurt Dressing:

- 4 oz (120 g) plain Greek yogurt
- 1 oz (30 ml) lemon juice
- 1 tbsp fresh parsley, chopped
- 1 tbsp fresh dill, chopped
- 1 tsp honey
- Salt and pepper to taste

Directions:

1. Preheat the oven to 400°F (200°C).
2. Toss the mixed vegetables with olive oil, salt, and pepper. Spread them on a baking sheet and roast for about 20-25 minutes, until they are tender and slightly caramelized.
3. In a large salad bowl, combine the mixed salad greens, cherry tomato halves, and thinly sliced red onion.
4. Top the salad with the roasted vegetables.
5. In a small bowl, mix together the plain Greek yogurt, lemon juice, chopped parsley, chopped dill, honey, salt, and pepper to make the herbed yogurt dressing.
6. Drizzle the herbed yogurt dressing over the salad.
7. Sprinkle the crumbled feta cheese on top.
8. Gently toss the salad to combine all the ingredients and coat them with the dressing.
9. Serve the roasted vegetable salad with herbed yogurt dressing as a delicious and nutritious meal.

Nutritional Values: Calories: 250 kcal | Fat: 16 g | Protein: 9 g | Carbs: 20 g | Net carbs: 15 g | Fiber: 5 g | Cholesterol: 20 mg | Sodium: 300 mg | Potassium: 650 mg

Useful Tip: Customize the vegetables in this recipe based on your preferences and what's in season. You can also add a sprinkle of toasted nuts or seeds for extra crunch and flavor.

Shrimp and Avocado Salad with Cilantro Lime Vinaigrette

Serving: 4 | Prep time: 20 minutes | Cook time: 5 minutes

Ingredients:

- 16 oz (450 g) large shrimp, peeled and deveined
- 1 tbsp olive oil
- Salt and pepper to taste
- 10 oz (280 g) mixed salad greens

- 2 avocados, diced
- 1 oz (150 g) cherry tomatoes, halved
- 1 oz (30 g) red onion, finely chopped

For Cilantro Lime Vinaigrette:

- 3 oz (90 ml) olive oil
- 1 oz (30 ml) lime juice
- 2 tbsp fresh cilantro, chopped

- 1 clove garlic, minced
- 1 tsp honey
- Salt and pepper to taste

Directions:

1. In a bowl, toss the shrimp with olive oil, salt, and pepper.
2. Heat a skillet over medium-high heat and cook the shrimp for about 2-3 minutes per side, until they are pink and cooked through. Set aside.
3. In a large salad bowl, combine the mixed salad greens, diced avocado, halved cherry tomatoes, and finely chopped red onion.
4. Top the salad with the cooked shrimp.
5. In a small bowl, whisk together olive oil, lime juice, chopped cilantro, minced garlic, honey, salt, and pepper to make the cilantro lime vinaigrette.
6. Drizzle the vinaigrette over the salad.
7. Gently toss the salad to combine all the ingredients and coat them with the vinaigrette.
8. Serve the shrimp and avocado salad with cilantro lime vinaigrette as a flavorful and satisfying meal.

Nutritional Values: Calories: 320 kcal | Fat: 25 g | Protein: 18 g | Carbs: 12 g | Net carbs: 7 g | Fiber: 5 g | Cholesterol: 160 mg | Sodium: 350 mg | Potassium: 750 mg

Useful Tip: You can customize this salad by adding other ingredients like toasted nuts, crumbled cheese, or sliced bell peppers for added texture and flavor.

Southwestern Black Bean and Corn Salad with Lime-Cilantro Dressing

Serving: 4 | Prep time: 15 minutes | Cook time: 0 minutes

Ingredients:

- 15 oz (425 g) canned black beans, drained and rinsed
- 8 oz (225 g) canned corn kernels, drained
- 1 red bell pepper, diced
- 1 avocado, diced

- 2 oz (60 g) red onion, finely chopped
- 2 oz (60 g) cherry tomatoes, halved
- 2 oz (60 g) fresh cilantro, chopped

For Lime-Cilantro Dressing:

- 3 oz (90 ml) olive oil
- 2 oz (60 ml) lime juice
- 1 tsp ground cumin

- 1 tsp chili powder
- Salt and pepper to taste

Directions:

1. In a large mixing bowl, combine the drained black beans, canned corn kernels, diced red bell pepper, diced avocado, finely chopped red onion, halved cherry tomatoes, and chopped fresh cilantro.
2. In a separate small bowl, whisk together the olive oil, lime juice, ground cumin, chili powder, salt, and pepper to create the lime-cilantro dressing.
3. Drizzle the dressing over the salad ingredients.
4. Gently toss the salad to ensure all ingredients are coated with the dressing.
5. Allow the flavors to meld for a few minutes before serving.
6. Serve the Southwestern black bean and corn salad with lime-cilantro dressing as a refreshing and nutritious dish.

Nutritional Values: Calories: 320 kcal | Fat: 18 g | Protein: 7 g | Carbs: 34 g | Net carbs: 25 g | Fiber: 9 g | Cholesterol: 0 mg | Sodium: 300 mg | Potassium: 700 mg

Useful Tip: For added protein, consider adding grilled chicken or cooked quinoa to make this salad a complete meal.

Roasted Cauliflower and Chickpea Salad with Turmeric Tahini

Serving: 4 | Prep time: 15 minutes | Cook time: 25 minutes

Ingredients:

- 16 oz (450 g) cauliflower florets
- 15 oz (425 g) canned chickpeas, drained and rinsed
- 2 oz (60 g) red onion, thinly sliced
- 2 oz (60 g) baby spinach leaves
- 1 oz (30 g) chopped fresh parsley
- 2 oz (60 ml) olive oil

For Turmeric Tahini Dressing:

- 3 oz (90 ml) tahini
- 2 oz (60 ml) water
- 1 oz (30 ml) lemon juice
- 1 tsp ground turmeric
- 1 tsp ground cumin
- Salt and pepper to taste

Directions:

1. Preheat the oven to 400°F (200°C).
2. In a large mixing bowl, combine the cauliflower florets and drained chickpeas. Toss with a drizzle of olive oil, salt, and pepper.
3. Spread the cauliflower and chickpeas on a baking sheet and roast in the preheated oven for about 20-25 minutes, or until the cauliflower is tender and golden brown.
4. While the cauliflower and chickpeas are roasting, prepare the turmeric tahini dressing by whisking together tahini, water, lemon juice, ground turmeric, ground cumin, salt, and pepper until smooth.
5. Once the cauliflower and chickpeas are roasted, remove them from the oven and let them cool slightly.
6. In a large salad bowl, combine the roasted cauliflower and chickpeas with thinly sliced red onion, baby spinach leaves, and chopped fresh parsley.
7. Drizzle the turmeric tahini dressing over the salad ingredients.
8. Gently toss the salad to ensure all ingredients are coated with the dressing.
9. Serve the roasted cauliflower and chickpea salad with turmeric tahini as a wholesome and flavorful dish.

Nutritional Values: Calories: 280 kcal | Fat: 18 g | Protein: 10 g | Carbs: 24 g | Net carbs: 16 g | Fiber: 8 g | Cholesterol: 0 mg | Sodium: 300 mg | Potassium: 800 mg

Useful Tip: Feel free to customize this salad by adding other vegetables like roasted red bell pepper or sliced cucumber.

Tuna Niçoise Salad with Lemon Herb Vinaigrette

Serving: 4 | Prep time: 20 minutes | Cook time: 15 minutes

Ingredients:

- 12 oz (340 g) canned tuna, drained
- 8 oz (225 g) green beans, blanched and cooled
- 4 oz (115 g) cherry tomatoes, halved
- 4 oz (115 g) baby potatoes, boiled and quartered
- 4 oz (115 g) mixed salad greens
- 2 oz (60 g) black olives
- 2 oz (60 g) red onion, thinly sliced
- 4 hard-boiled eggs, halved

For Lemon Herb Vinaigrette:

- 2 oz (60 ml) olive oil
- 1 oz (30 ml) lemon juice
- 1 tsp Dijon mustard
- 1 tbsp chopped fresh parsley
- 1 tbsp chopped fresh basil
- Salt and pepper to taste

Directions:

1. In a large salad bowl, arrange the mixed salad greens as the base.
2. Arrange the blanched green beans, cherry tomatoes, boiled baby potatoes, black olives, red onion, and hard-boiled eggs on top of the salad greens.
3. In a small bowl, whisk together the ingredients for the lemon herb vinaigrette: olive oil, lemon juice, Dijon mustard, chopped parsley, chopped basil, salt, and pepper.
4. Drizzle the lemon herb vinaigrette over the salad ingredients.
5. Flake the canned tuna and distribute it over the salad.
6. Serve the Tuna Niçoise Salad with Lemon Herb Vinaigrette as a nourishing and delicious meal.

Nutritional Values: Calories: 350 kcal | Fat: 25 g | Protein: 20 g | Carbs: 15 g | Net carbs: 10 g | Fiber: 5 g | Cholesterol: 160 mg | Sodium: 450 mg | Potassium: 600 mg

Useful Tip: For extra flavor, marinate the canned tuna with a bit of lemon juice and olive oil before adding it to the salad.

Moroccan Couscous Salad with Roasted Vegetables and Harissa Dressing

Serving: 4 | Prep time: 15 minutes | Cook time: 25 minutes

Ingredients:

- 8 oz (225 g) couscous
- 12 oz (340 g) mixed vegetables (bell peppers, zucchini, eggplant), chopped
- 2 oz (60 g) red onion, thinly sliced

- 4 oz (115 g) cherry tomatoes, halved
- 4 oz (115 g) canned chickpeas, drained and rinsed
- 2 oz (60 g) raisins
- 2 oz (60 g) toasted almonds, chopped

For Harissa Dressing:

- 3 oz (90 ml) olive oil
- 1 oz (30 ml) lemon juice
- 1 tbsp harissa paste

- 1 tsp ground cumin
- Salt and pepper to taste
- Fresh cilantro leaves for garnish

Directions:

1. Cook the couscous according to package instructions, fluff with a fork, and set aside to cool.
2. Preheat the oven to 400°F (200°C).
3. Toss the chopped mixed vegetables with a drizzle of olive oil, salt, and pepper, and spread them on a baking sheet. Roast in the preheated oven for about 20-25 minutes or until they are tender and slightly caramelized.
4. In a large bowl, combine the cooked couscous, roasted vegetables, sliced red onion, halved cherry tomatoes, canned chickpeas, and raisins.
5. In a small bowl, whisk together the ingredients for the harissa dressing: olive oil, lemon juice, harissa paste, ground cumin, salt, and pepper.
6. Drizzle the harissa dressing over the couscous mixture and toss well to coat.
7. Sprinkle the toasted almonds over the top and garnish with fresh cilantro leaves.
8. Serve the Moroccan Couscous Salad with Roasted Vegetables and Harissa Dressing as a flavorful and satisfying meal.

Nutritional Values: Calories: 380 kcal | Fat: 18 g | Protein: 8 g | Carbs: 50 g | Net carbs: 42 g | Fiber: 8 g | Cholesterol: 0 mg | Sodium: 320 mg | Potassium: 600 mg

Useful Tip: You can customize this salad by adding grilled chicken, roasted shrimp, or crumbled feta cheese for extra protein and flavor.

Roasted Brussels Sprouts and Quinoa Salad with Lemon Mustard Dressing

Serving: 4 | Prep time: 15 minutes | Cook time: 25 minutes

Ingredients:

- 8 oz (225 g) Brussels sprouts, trimmed and halved
- 5 oz (140 g) quinoa
- 2 oz (60 g) red onion, finely chopped

- 2 oz (60 g) dried cranberries
- 2 oz (60 g) chopped pecans

For Lemon Mustard Dressing:

- 3 oz (90 ml) olive oil
- 1 oz (30 ml) lemon juice
- 1 tsp Dijon mustard

- 1 tsp honey
- Salt and pepper to taste
- Fresh parsley leaves for garnish

Directions:

1. Preheat the oven to 400°F (200°C).
2. Toss the halved Brussels sprouts with a drizzle of olive oil, salt, and pepper, and spread them on a baking sheet. Roast in the preheated oven for about 20-25 minutes or until they are tender and crispy.
3. Cook the quinoa according to package instructions, fluff with a fork, and let it cool.
4. In a large bowl, combine the cooked quinoa, roasted Brussels sprouts, finely chopped red onion, dried cranberries, and chopped pecans.
5. In a small bowl, whisk together the ingredients for the lemon mustard dressing: olive oil, lemon juice, Dijon mustard, honey, salt, and pepper.
6. Drizzle the lemon mustard dressing over the quinoa and Brussels sprouts mixture and toss well to coat.
7. Garnish the salad with fresh parsley leaves.
8. Serve the Roasted Brussels Sprouts and Quinoa Salad with Lemon Mustard Dressing as a nutritious and delicious meal.

Nutritional Values: Calories: 360 kcal | Fat: 20 g | Protein: 7 g | Carbs: 40 g | Net carbs: 32 g | Fiber: 8 g | Cholesterol: 0 mg | Sodium: 120 mg | Potassium: 530 mg

Useful Tip: For added protein, you can top this salad with grilled chicken, roasted chickpeas, or crumbled feta cheese.

Mexican Street Corn Salad with Chili Lime Dressing

Serving: 4 | Prep time: 15 minutes | Cook time: 10 minutes

Ingredients:

- 16 oz (450 g) frozen corn kernels, thawed
- 2 oz (60 g) red onion, finely chopped
- 2 oz (60 g) cotija cheese, crumbled
- 2 tbsp mayonnaise
- 2 tbsp fresh lime juice
- 1 tsp chili powder
- 1 tsp smoked paprika
- 1/2 tsp cayenne pepper (adjust to taste)
- Salt and black pepper to taste
- 0.25 oz (15 g) fresh cilantro, chopped
- Lime wedges for garnish

Directions:

1. Heat a skillet over medium-high heat and add the thawed corn kernels. Cook for about 5-7 minutes or until the corn is slightly charred.
2. In a large bowl, combine the cooked corn, finely chopped red onion, and crumbled cotija cheese.
3. In a separate small bowl, whisk together the mayonnaise, fresh lime juice, chili powder, smoked paprika, cayenne pepper, salt, and black pepper to make the chili lime dressing.
4. Pour the chili lime dressing over the corn mixture and toss to combine, ensuring everything is well coated.
5. Sprinkle the chopped cilantro over the salad and gently toss again.
6. Garnish the Mexican Street Corn Salad with Lime wedges for an extra burst of flavor.
7. Serve this delicious and vibrant salad as a side dish or light meal option.

Nutritional Values: Calories: 220 kcal | Fat: 12 g | Protein: 6 g | Carbs: 25 g | Net carbs: 20 g | Fiber: 5 g | Cholesterol: 20 mg | Sodium: 320 mg | Potassium: 390 mg

Useful Tip: For a twist, you can add some diced avocado or grilled chicken to make it heartier and more substantial.

Roasted Butternut Squash and Pomegranate Salad with Maple Dijon Dressing

Serving: 4 | Prep time: 15 minutes | Cook time: 25 minutes

Ingredients:

- 24 oz (680 g) butternut squash, peeled, seeded, and cubed
- 2 oz (60 ml) olive oil
- Salt and black pepper to taste
- 4 oz (115 g) baby spinach or mixed greens
- 1 pomegranate, seeds removed
- 2 oz (60 g) walnuts, toasted and chopped
- 2 oz (60 g) goat cheese, crumbled

For Maple Dijon Dressing:

- 1 oz (30 ml) olive oil
- 1 oz (30 ml) apple cider vinegar
- 0.5 oz (15 ml) maple syrup
- 1 tsp Dijon mustard
- Salt and black pepper to taste

Directions:

1. Preheat the oven to 400°F (200°C).
2. Toss the cubed butternut squash with olive oil, salt, and black pepper in a bowl.
3. Spread the butternut squash on a baking sheet in a single layer and roast in the preheated oven for about 20-25 minutes or until tender and slightly caramelized.
4. In a large bowl, combine the roasted butternut squash, baby spinach or mixed greens, pomegranate seeds, toasted walnuts, and crumbled goat cheese.
5. In a small bowl, whisk together the olive oil, apple cider vinegar, maple syrup, Dijon mustard, salt, and black pepper to make the maple Dijon dressing.
6. Drizzle the dressing over the salad and toss gently to combine.
7. Serve the Roasted Butternut Squash and Pomegranate Salad with Maple Dijon Dressing as a delicious and nutritious meal.

Nutritional Values: Calories: 320 kcal | Fat: 22 g | Protein: 6 g | Carbs: 29 g | Net carbs: 22 g | Fiber: 7 g | Cholesterol: 10 mg | Sodium: 220 mg | Potassium: 650 mg

Useful Tip: To easily remove pomegranate seeds, cut the pomegranate in half and gently tap the back of each half with a wooden spoon to release the seeds.

Grilled Chicken Caesar Salad with Creamy Avocado Dressing

Serving: 4 | Prep time: 15 minutes | Cook time: 15 minutes

Ingredients:

- 16 oz (450 g) boneless, skinless chicken breasts
- 1 oz (30 ml) olive oil
- Salt and black pepper to taste

- 8 oz (225 g) romaine lettuce, washed and chopped
- 2 oz (60 g) grated Parmesan cheese
- 2 oz (60 g) whole wheat croutons

For Creamy Avocado Dressing:

- 1 ripe avocado, peeled and pitted
- 2 oz (60 ml) plain Greek yogurt
- 1 oz (30 ml) lemon juice

- 1 garlic clove, minced
- 1 tsp Dijon mustard
- Salt and black pepper to taste

Directions:

1. Preheat the grill to medium-high heat.
2. Rub the chicken breasts with olive oil, salt, and black pepper.
3. Grill the chicken breasts for about 6-8 minutes per side or until they are cooked through and have nice grill marks. Remove from the grill and let them rest for a few minutes before slicing.
4. In a blender or food processor, combine the avocado, Greek yogurt, lemon juice, minced garlic, Dijon mustard, salt, and black pepper. Blend until smooth to make the creamy avocado dressing.
5. In a large bowl, toss the chopped romaine lettuce with the creamy avocado dressing.
6. Divide the dressed lettuce among serving plates.
7. Top each plate with sliced grilled chicken, grated Parmesan cheese, and whole wheat croutons.
8. Serve the Grilled Chicken Caesar Salad with Creamy Avocado Dressing as a satisfying and nutritious meal.

Nutritional Values: Calories: 330 kcal | Fat: 15 g | Protein: 35 g | Carbs: 15 g | Net carbs: 10 g | Fiber: 5 g | Cholesterol: 80 mg | Sodium: 420 mg | Potassium: 700 mg

Useful Tip: To make homemade whole wheat croutons, cut whole wheat bread into cubes, toss with olive oil and your favorite herbs, then bake in the oven until crispy.

Roasted Eggplant and Tomato Salad with Balsamic Glaze

Serving: 4 | Prep time: 15 minutes | Cook time: 20 minutes

Ingredients:

- 1 medium eggplant, cut into 1-inch cubes
- 8 oz (225 g) cherry tomatoes, halved
- 2 oz (60 ml) olive oil
- Salt and black pepper to taste

- 2 oz (60 g) red onion, thinly sliced
- 2 oz (60 g) crumbled feta cheese
- Fresh basil leaves for garnish

For Balsamic Glaze:

- 2 oz (60 ml) balsamic vinegar
- 1 oz honey

- 1 tsp olive oil

Directions:

1. Preheat the oven to 400°F (200°C).
2. Place the eggplant cubes on a baking sheet and drizzle with olive oil. Season with salt and black pepper, then toss to coat.
3. Roast the eggplant in the preheated oven for about 15-20 minutes, or until golden and tender. Stir once halfway through.
4. While the eggplant is roasting, prepare the balsamic glaze. In a small saucepan, combine the balsamic vinegar and honey. Bring to a simmer over medium heat and cook for about 5-7 minutes, or until the mixture has reduced by half and has a syrupy consistency. Remove from heat and stir in the teaspoon of olive oil.
5. In a large bowl, combine the roasted eggplant, cherry tomatoes, and thinly sliced red onion.
6. Drizzle the balsamic glaze over the salad and gently toss to combine.
7. Transfer the salad to serving plates, and sprinkle crumbled feta cheese over the top.
8. Garnish with fresh basil leaves for an added burst of flavor and freshness.

Nutritional Values: Calories: 220 kcal | Fat: 14 g | Protein: 4 g | Carbs: 22 g | Net carbs: 18 g | Fiber: 4 g | Cholesterol: 15 mg | Sodium: 270 mg | Potassium: 480 mg

Useful Tip: To prevent the eggplant from becoming too mushy when roasting, you can sprinkle the eggplant cubes with salt and let them sit for about 15 minutes before roasting. Rinse and pat dry before roasting.

Creamy Broccoli and Cauliflower Soup with Garlic Parmesan Croutons

Serving: 4 | Prep time: 15 minutes | Cook time: 25 minutes

Ingredients:

- 8 oz (225 g) broccoli florets
- 8 oz (225 g) cauliflower florets
- 2 oz (60 g) onion, chopped
- 2 cloves garlic, minced
- 1 oz (30 ml) olive oil

- 32 oz (960 ml) vegetable broth
- 2 oz (60 ml) unsweetened almond milk
- Salt and black pepper to taste
- 2 oz (60 g) grated Parmesan cheese

For Garlic Parmesan Croutons:

- 2 oz (60 g) whole grain bread, cubed
- 1 tbsp olive oil
- 1 clove garlic, minced

- 1 oz (30 g) grated Parmesan cheese
- Fresh parsley for garnish

Directions:

1. In a large pot, heat the olive oil over medium heat. Add the chopped onion and minced garlic, and sauté until the onion becomes translucent.
2. Add the broccoli and cauliflower florets to the pot, and sauté for a few minutes to enhance their flavors.
3. Pour in the vegetable broth and bring to a simmer. Cover and cook for about 15-20 minutes, or until the vegetables are tender.
4. Use an immersion blender to carefully blend the soup until smooth and creamy.
5. Stir in the unsweetened almond milk and grated Parmesan cheese. Season with salt and black pepper to taste.
6. For the Garlic Parmesan Croutons, preheat the oven to 350°F (175°C). In a bowl, toss the bread cubes with olive oil, minced garlic, and grated Parmesan cheese. Spread the cubes on a baking sheet and bake for about 10-12 minutes, or until golden and crispy.
7. Ladle the creamy soup into serving bowls and garnish with a handful of Garlic Parmesan Croutons and fresh parsley.

Nutritional Values: Calories: 280 kcal | Fat: 15 g | Protein: 12 g | Carbs: 26 g | Net carbs: 20 g | Fiber: 6 g | Cholesterol: 20 mg | Sodium: 700 mg | Potassium: 700 mg

Useful Tip: To make the soup even creamier, you can add a small boiled and peeled potato to the pot before blending.

Spiced Lentil and Vegetable Soup with Turmeric Yogurt Drizzle

Serving: 4 | Prep time: 15 minutes | Cook time: 30 minutes

Ingredients:

- 4 oz (115 g) dried green or brown lentils, rinsed and drained
- 2 oz (60 g) onion, chopped
- 2 oz (60 g) carrots, peeled and diced
- 2 oz (60 g) celery, diced
- 2 cloves garlic, minced
- 1 oz (30 ml) olive oil
- 32 oz (960 ml) vegetable broth

- 14 oz (400 g) canned diced tomatoes
- 1 tsp ground cumin
- 1 tsp ground coriander
- 1/2 tsp ground turmeric
- 1/4 tsp cayenne pepper (adjust to taste)
- Salt and black pepper to taste
- Fresh cilantro leaves for garnish

For Turmeric Yogurt Drizzle:

- 4 oz (120 g) plain Greek yogurt
- 1/2 tsp ground turmeric

- 1 tsp lemon juice
- Salt to taste

Directions:

1. In a large pot, heat the olive oil over medium heat. Add the chopped onion, diced carrots, diced celery, and minced garlic. Sauté for a few minutes until the vegetables start to soften.
2. Add the ground cumin, ground coriander, ground turmeric, and cayenne pepper to the pot. Stir well to coat the vegetables in the spices.
3. Add the rinsed lentils, vegetable broth, and canned diced tomatoes to the pot. Bring to a boil, then reduce the heat and let it simmer for about 20-25 minutes, or until the lentils are tender.

4. Use an immersion blender to blend a portion of the soup to create a thicker consistency while still leaving some chunks.
5. Season the soup with salt and black pepper to taste.
6. In a small bowl, mix together the plain Greek yogurt, ground turmeric, lemon juice, and a pinch of salt to make the Turmeric Yogurt Drizzle.
7. Ladle the spiced lentil and vegetable soup into serving bowls, drizzle with the Turmeric Yogurt, and garnish with fresh cilantro leaves.

Nutritional Values: Calories: 250 kcal | Fat: 8 g | Protein: 12 g | Carbs: 36 g | Net carbs: 28 g | Fiber: 8 g | Cholesterol: 10 mg | Sodium: 800 mg | Potassium: 800 mg

Useful Tip: For added protein, you can stir in some cooked quinoa or serve the soup with a side of whole grain bread.

Thai Coconut Chicken Soup with Lemongrass and Lime

Serving: 4 | Prep time: 15 minutes | Cook time: 25 minutes

Ingredients:

- 12 oz (340 g) boneless, skinless chicken breast, thinly sliced
- 2 oz (60 g) onion, finely chopped
- 2 cloves garlic, minced
- 1 oz (30 ml) coconut oil
- 1 stalk lemongrass, smashed and cut into 2-inch pieces
- 1 thumb-sized piece of ginger, sliced
- 3 oz (90 g) mushrooms, sliced
- 2 oz (60 g) red bell pepper, thinly sliced

- 1 oz (30 g) Thai red curry paste
- 32 oz (960 ml) chicken broth
- 14 oz (400 ml) canned coconut milk
- 1 lime, zested and juiced
- 1 tbsp fish sauce
- 1 tsp brown sugar
- Fresh cilantro leaves for garnish
- Sliced red chili peppers for garnish (optional)

Directions:

1. In a large pot, heat the coconut oil over medium heat. Add the chopped onion and minced garlic. Sauté until the onion is translucent.
2. Add the Thai red curry paste and cook for a minute until fragrant.
3. Add the sliced chicken breast to the pot and cook until no longer pink.
4. Add the sliced mushrooms and red bell pepper to the pot and sauté for a few minutes until they start to soften.
5. Pour in the chicken broth and canned coconut milk. Add the smashed lemongrass and sliced ginger.
6. Bring the soup to a gentle simmer and let it cook for about 15 minutes to allow the flavors to meld.
7. Stir in the lime zest, lime juice, fish sauce, and brown sugar. Adjust the seasoning according to taste.
8. Remove the lemongrass pieces and ginger slices from the soup.
9. Ladle the Thai Coconut Chicken Soup into serving bowls, garnish with fresh cilantro leaves and sliced red chili peppers if desired.

Nutritional Values: Calories: 280 kcal | Fat: 15 g | Protein: 25 g | Carbs: 14 g | Net carbs: 10 g | Fiber: 4 g | Cholesterol: 60 mg | Sodium: 900 mg | Potassium: 600 mg

Useful Tip: If you prefer a spicier soup, you can add some extra Thai red curry paste or sliced red chili peppers.

Roasted Red Pepper and Tomato Soup with Basil Pesto Swirl

Serving: 4 | Prep time: 15 minutes | Cook time: 30 minutes

Ingredients:

- 2 large red bell peppers, halved and seeds removed
- 14 oz (400 g) canned diced tomatoes
- 1 oz (30 ml) olive oil
- 1 oz (30 g) onion, chopped
- 2 cloves garlic, minced
- 32 oz (960 ml) vegetable broth
- 1 tsp dried basil
- 1 tsp dried oregano
- Salt and pepper to taste
- 2 oz (60 ml) unsweetened almond milk
- 2 oz (60 g) fresh basil leaves
- 1 oz (30 g) pine nuts
- 1 oz (30 g) grated Parmesan cheese
- 1 oz (30 ml) olive oil (for pesto)
- 1 oz (30 g) sun-dried tomatoes (for pesto)

Directions:

1. Preheat the oven to 400°F (200°C). Place the red bell pepper halves on a baking sheet, skin side up. Roast in the oven until the skins are charred and blistered, about 20 minutes. Remove from the oven, cover with a kitchen towel, and let them cool. Once cooled, peel off the skins and chop the roasted peppers.
2. In a large pot, heat the olive oil over medium heat. Add the chopped onion and minced garlic. Sauté until the onion is translucent.
3. Add the chopped roasted red peppers, canned diced tomatoes, vegetable broth, dried basil, dried oregano, salt, and pepper to the pot. Let the soup simmer for about 15 minutes.
4. Use an immersion blender to puree the soup until smooth. Stir in the unsweetened almond milk and let the soup heat through.
5. In a food processor, combine the fresh basil leaves, pine nuts, grated Parmesan cheese, olive oil, and sun-dried tomatoes. Blend until a smooth pesto mixture forms.
6. Ladle the Roasted Red Pepper and Tomato Soup into serving bowls and drizzle each portion with a swirl of basil pesto.

Nutritional Values: Calories: 220 kcal | Fat: 15 g | Protein: 6 g | Carbs: 18 g | Net carbs: 13 g | Fiber: 5 g | Cholesterol: 5 mg | Sodium: 800 mg | Potassium: 600 mg

Useful Tip: To make the basil pesto more flavorful, lightly toast the pine nuts in a dry skillet over medium heat before blending.

Hearty Mushroom and Barley Soup with Fresh Thyme

Serving: 4 | Prep time: 15 minutes | Cook time: 40 minutes

Ingredients:

- 8 oz (225 g) mushrooms, sliced
- 4 oz (115 g) carrots, diced
- 4 oz (115 g) celery, diced
- 2 oz (60 g) onion, chopped
- 2 cloves garlic, minced
- 1 oz (30 ml) olive oil
- 2 oz (60 g) pearl barley
- 32 oz (960 ml) vegetable broth
- 1 tsp fresh thyme leaves
- Salt and pepper to taste
- 2 oz (60 ml) unsweetened almond milk
- 1 oz (30 g) fresh thyme sprigs (for garnish)

Directions:

1. In a large pot, heat the olive oil over medium heat. Add the chopped onion and minced garlic. Sauté until the onion is translucent.
2. Add the diced carrots and celery to the pot and sauté for another 5 minutes until they start to soften.
3. Stir in the sliced mushrooms and pearl barley. Cook for a few more minutes until the mushrooms release their moisture.
4. Pour in the vegetable broth and add the fresh thyme leaves. Season with salt and pepper to taste. Bring the soup to a boil, then reduce the heat to low and let it simmer for about 30 minutes until the barley is tender.
5. Stir in the unsweetened almond milk to add creaminess to the soup.
6. Ladle the Hearty Mushroom and Barley Soup into serving bowls and garnish with fresh thyme sprigs.

Nutritional Values: Calories: 250 kcal | Fat: 7 g | Protein: 5 g | Carbs: 42 g | Net carbs: 36 g | Fiber: 6 g | Cholesterol: 0 mg | Sodium: 700 mg | Potassium: 600 mg

Useful Tip: For extra depth of flavor, you can sauté the mushrooms separately in a dry skillet until they are browned and slightly caramelized before adding them to the soup.

Butternut Squash and Carrot Soup with Toasted Pumpkin Seeds

Serving: 4 | Prep time: 15 minutes | Cook time: 30 minutes

Ingredients:

- 16 oz (450 g) butternut squash, peeled and diced
- 8 oz (225 g) carrots, peeled and sliced
- 2 oz (60 g) onion, chopped
- 2 cloves garlic, minced
- 1 oz (30 ml) olive oil
- 32 oz (960 ml) vegetable broth
- 1 tsp ground cumin
- 1/2 tsp ground cinnamon
- Salt and pepper to taste
- 2 oz (60 ml) coconut milk
- 2 oz (60 g) pumpkin seeds, toasted
- Fresh cilantro leaves (for garnish)

Directions:

1. In a large pot, heat the olive oil over medium heat. Add the chopped onion and minced garlic. Sauté until the onion is translucent.
2. Add the diced butternut squash and sliced carrots to the pot. Sauté for a few minutes until they start to soften.
3. Stir in the ground cumin and ground cinnamon. Season with salt and pepper to taste.
4. Pour in the vegetable broth and bring the soup to a boil. Reduce the heat to low and let it simmer for about 20-25 minutes, or until the vegetables are tender.
5. Use an immersion blender to puree the soup until smooth and creamy.
6. Stir in the coconut milk to add richness to the soup.
7. Ladle the Butternut Squash and Carrot Soup into serving bowls and garnish with toasted pumpkin seeds and fresh cilantro leaves.

Nutritional Values: Calories: 180 kcal | Fat: 10 g | Protein: 5 g | Carbs: 20 g | Net carbs: 16 g | Fiber: 4 g | Cholesterol: 0 mg | Sodium: 700 mg | Potassium: 800 mg

Useful Tip: To toast pumpkin seeds, heat a dry skillet over medium heat. Add the pumpkin seeds and cook, stirring frequently, until they are golden brown and start to pop. Be careful not to burn them.

Moroccan Spiced Chickpea Soup with Harissa Yogurt Dollop

Serving: 4 | Prep time: 15 minutes | Cook time: 30 minutes

Ingredients:

- 16 oz (450 g) canned chickpeas, drained and rinsed
- 2 oz (60 g) onion, chopped
- 2 cloves garlic, minced
- 2 oz (60 g) carrot, diced
- 2 oz (60 g) celery, diced
- 1 oz (30 ml) olive oil
- 1 tsp ground cumin
- 1/2 tsp ground coriander
- 1/2 tsp ground turmeric
- 1/4 tsp ground cinnamon
- Pinch of cayenne pepper (adjust to taste)
- 32 oz (960 ml) vegetable broth
- Salt and pepper to taste
- 2 oz (60 ml) plain Greek yogurt
- 1 tsp harissa paste
- Fresh cilantro leaves (for garnish)

Directions:

1. In a large pot, heat the olive oil over medium heat. Add the chopped onion and minced garlic. Sauté until the onion is translucent.
2. Add the diced carrot and celery to the pot. Sauté for a few minutes until they start to soften.
3. Stir in the ground cumin, ground coriander, ground turmeric, ground cinnamon, and cayenne pepper. Season with salt and pepper to taste.
4. Add the canned chickpeas to the pot and mix well to coat them with the spices.
5. Pour in the vegetable broth and bring the soup to a boil. Reduce the heat to low and let it simmer for about 20-25 minutes.
6. While the soup is simmering, mix the plain Greek yogurt with harissa paste to create the harissa yogurt dollop.
7. Use an immersion blender to puree a portion of the soup to create a creamy texture while leaving some chickpeas whole.
8. Ladle the Moroccan Spiced Chickpea Soup into serving bowls and top each bowl with a dollop of harissa yogurt and fresh cilantro leaves.

Nutritional Values: Calories: 220 kcal | Fat: 6 g | Protein: 9 g | Carbs: 33 g | Net carbs: 26 g | Fiber: 7 g | Cholesterol: 0 mg | Sodium: 800 mg | Potassium: 600 mg

Useful Tip: Harissa paste can vary in spiciness, so start with a small amount and adjust to your taste preference.

Creamy Spinach and White Bean Soup with Lemon Zest

Serving: 4 | Prep time: 10 minutes | Cook time: 25 minutes

Ingredients:

- 8 oz (225 g) fresh spinach, chopped
- 15 oz (425 g) canned white beans, drained and rinsed
- 2 oz (60 g) onion, chopped
- 2 cloves garlic, minced
- 2 oz (60 g) celery, diced
- 1 oz (30 ml) olive oil
- 32 oz (960 ml) vegetable broth
- 1 tsp dried thyme
- 1/2 tsp ground nutmeg
- Zest of 1 lemon
- 4 oz (120 ml) unsweetened almond milk
- Salt and pepper to taste
- Fresh parsley leaves (for garnish)

Directions:

1. In a large pot, heat the olive oil over medium heat. Add the chopped onion and minced garlic. Sauté until the onion is translucent.
2. Add the diced celery to the pot and sauté for a few minutes until it starts to soften.
3. Stir in the chopped spinach and cook until wilted.
4. Add the canned white beans, dried thyme, ground nutmeg, and lemon zest to the pot. Season with salt and pepper to taste.
5. Pour in the vegetable broth and bring the soup to a boil. Reduce the heat to low and let it simmer for about 15-20 minutes.
6. Use an immersion blender to blend a portion of the soup until creamy while leaving some chunks of white beans and vegetables.
7. Stir in the unsweetened almond milk to add creaminess to the soup.
8. Ladle the Creamy Spinach and White Bean Soup into serving bowls and garnish with fresh parsley leaves.

Nutritional Values: Calories: 190 kcal | Fat: 6 g | Protein: 10 g | Carbs: 26 g | Net carbs: 20 g | Fiber: 6 g | Cholesterol: 0 mg | Sodium: 800 mg | Potassium: 700 mg

Useful Tip: For an extra burst of lemon flavor, you can squeeze some fresh lemon juice into the soup before serving.

Zesty Gazpacho with Avocado and Cilantro Garnish

Serving: 4 | Prep time: 15 minutes | Cook time: 0 minutes

Ingredients:

- 28 oz (800 g) canned whole tomatoes, drained
- 1 cucumber, peeled and diced
- 1 red bell pepper, diced
- 1 small red onion, diced
- 2 cloves garlic, minced
- 2 oz (60 ml) olive oil
- 2 oz (60 ml) red wine vinegar
- 1 tsp cumin
- 1/2 tsp smoked paprika
- 1/2 tsp cayenne pepper
- Salt and pepper to taste
- 1 ripe avocado, diced (for garnish)
- Fresh cilantro leaves (for garnish)

Directions:

1. In a blender, combine the canned whole tomatoes, diced cucumber, diced red bell pepper, diced red onion, minced garlic, olive oil, red wine vinegar, cumin, smoked paprika, cayenne pepper, salt, and pepper.
2. Blend until the mixture is smooth and well combined.
3. Taste and adjust the seasoning if needed by adding more salt, pepper, or spices.
4. Chill the gazpacho in the refrigerator for at least 1 hour to allow the flavors to meld together.
5. To serve, ladle the chilled gazpacho into bowls and garnish with diced avocado and fresh cilantro leaves.

Nutritional Values: Calories: 160 kcal | Fat: 11 g | Protein: 2 g | Carbs: 15 g | Net carbs: 10 g | Fiber: 5 g | Cholesterol: 0 mg | Sodium: 400 mg | Potassium: 600 mg

Useful Tip: For a creamier texture, you can add a dollop of Greek yogurt or a splash of unsweetened almond milk to each bowl before serving.

Turkey and Vegetable Quinoa Soup with Herbed Quinoa Topping

Serving: 4 | Prep time: 15 minutes | Cook time: 30 minutes

Ingredients:

- 8 oz (225 g) lean ground turkey
- 1 small onion, finely chopped
- 2 carrots, diced
- 2 celery stalks, diced
- 2 cloves garlic, minced
- 1 zucchini, diced
- 2 tbsp chopped fresh basil
- 32 oz (900 ml) low-sodium chicken or vegetable broth
- 1 red bell pepper, diced
- 1 tsp dried thyme
- 1 tsp dried oregano
- Salt and pepper to taste
- 4 oz (115 g) cooked quinoa
- 2 tbsp chopped fresh parsley
- 14 oz (400 g) canned diced tomatoes
- 1 tbsp olive oil

Directions:

1. In a large pot, brown the lean ground turkey over medium heat until cooked through. Remove any excess fat.
2. Add the chopped onion, diced carrots, diced celery, and minced garlic to the pot. Sauté for 5 minutes until the vegetables begin to soften.
3. Stir in the diced zucchini and diced red bell pepper and cook for an additional 3 minutes.
4. Pour in the low-sodium chicken or vegetable broth and canned diced tomatoes. Add dried thyme and dried oregano. Season with salt and pepper to taste.
5. Bring the soup to a boil, then reduce the heat and let it simmer for about 15 minutes, allowing the flavors to meld together.
6. In a small bowl, combine the cooked quinoa with chopped fresh parsley and basil. Drizzle with olive oil and mix well.
7. To serve, ladle the soup into bowls and top each bowl with a spoonful of the herbed quinoa mixture.

Nutritional Values: Calories: 220 kcal | Fat: 7 g | Protein: 16 g | Carbs: 25 g | Net carbs: 20 g | Fiber: 5 g | Cholesterol: 35 mg | Sodium: 600 mg | Potassium: 800 mg

Useful Tip: You can make the herbed quinoa topping in advance and store it separately to sprinkle on each serving of soup right before enjoying.

Chapter 6. Vegan Recipes

Roasted Vegetable Quinoa Bowl with Lemon-Tahini Dressing

Serving: 4 | Prep time: 15 minutes | Cook time: 25 minutes

Ingredients:

- 8 oz (225 g) mixed vegetables (e.g., bell peppers, zucchini, and carrots), chopped
- 2 oz (60 ml) olive oil
- 0.5 tsp salt
- 0.25 tsp black pepper
- 1 oz (180 g) quinoa, rinsed
- 16 oz (475 ml) water
- 2 oz (60 ml) lemon juice
- 3 tbsp tahini
- 2 cloves garlic, minced
- 0.25 tsp cumin
- 0.25 tsp paprika
- 2 tbsp chopped fresh parsley

Directions:

1. Preheat the oven to 400°F (200°C).
2. In a mixing bowl, toss the chopped mixed vegetables with 1 ounce of olive oil, salt, and black pepper. Spread them evenly on a baking sheet and roast in the preheated oven for 20-25 minutes or until the vegetables are tender and slightly caramelized.
3. While the vegetables are roasting, rinse the quinoa thoroughly under cold water. In a saucepan, combine the rinsed quinoa and 16 ounces of water. Bring to a boil, then reduce the heat to low, cover, and let it simmer for 15 minutes or until the quinoa is cooked and the water is absorbed. Fluff the quinoa with a fork.
4. In a small bowl, whisk together the remaining 1 ounce of olive oil, lemon juice, tahini, minced garlic, cumin, and paprika to make the dressing.
5. To assemble the bowls, divide the cooked quinoa among 4 serving bowls. Top each bowl with the roasted vegetables and drizzle with the lemon-tahini dressing.
6. Sprinkle chopped fresh parsley over the bowls for an extra burst of flavor.
7. Enjoy the dish.

Nutritional Values: Calories: 320 kcal | Fat: 15 g | Protein: 9 g | Carbs: 38 g | Net carbs: 31 g | Fiber: 7 g | Cholesterol: 0 mg | Sodium: 380 mg | Potassium: 582 mg

Useful Tip: Feel free to customize this bowl with your favorite roasted vegetables and adjust the seasoning to your taste preferences.

Spicy Chickpea and Spinach Curry with Fragrant Basmati Rice

Serving: 4 | Prep time: 10 minutes | Cook time: 25 minutes

Ingredients:

- 14 oz (400 g) canned chickpeas, drained and rinsed
- 8 oz (225 g) fresh spinach, washed and chopped
- 2 tbsp olive oil
- 1 large onion, finely chopped
- 2 cloves garlic, minced
- 1 tsp ginger, grated
- 1 tbsp curry powder
- 1/2 tsp ground cumin
- 1/2 tsp ground coriander
- 1/4 tsp cayenne pepper (adjust to taste)
- 14 oz (400 g) canned diced tomatoes
- 8 oz (240 ml) vegetable broth
- Salt to taste
- 8 oz (225 g) basmati rice
- 16 oz (475 ml) water
- Fresh cilantro leaves for garnish

Directions:

1. In a large pot, heat the olive oil over medium heat.
2. Add the chopped onion, minced garlic, and grated ginger. Sauté until the onion is translucent.
3. Stir in the curry powder, ground cumin, ground coriander, and cayenne pepper. Cook for about 1-2 minutes to release the spices' flavors.
4. Add the drained chickpeas, diced tomatoes, and vegetable broth. Season with salt to taste. Simmer the mixture for 10-15 minutes, allowing the flavors to meld and the sauce to thicken.
5. While the curry is simmering, rinse the basmati rice under cold water until the water runs clear. In a separate pot, combine the rinsed rice and 16 ounces of water. Bring to a boil, then reduce the heat to low, cover, and let it simmer for about 15-18 minutes or until the rice is cooked and the water is absorbed.
6. When the rice is cooked, fluff it with a fork and cover to keep warm.
7. Just before serving, stir in the chopped spinach into the chickpea curry and cook until wilted.
8. Serve the spicy chickpea and spinach curry over fragrant basmati rice, garnished with fresh cilantro leaves.
9. Enjoy the dish.

Nutritional Values: Calories: 380 kcal | Fat: 8 g | Protein: 10 g | Carbs: 67 g | Net carbs: 56 g | Fiber: 11 g | Cholesterol: 0 mg | Sodium: 720 mg | Potassium: 960 mg

Useful Tip: For a creamier curry, you can add a splash of coconut milk or a dollop of yogurt before serving.

Zucchini Noodles with Creamy Avocado Pesto and Cherry Tomatoes

Serving: 4 | Prep time: 15 minutes | Cook time: 5 minutes

Ingredients:

- 4 medium zucchinis, spiralized into noodles (about 16 oz / 450 g)
- 2 ripe avocados, peeled and pitted
- 10 oz (300 g) cherry tomatoes, halved
- 1 oz (30 ml) olive oil
- 1 oz (30 ml) water
- 0.5 oz (15 g) fresh basil leaves
- 0.5 oz (15 g) fresh parsley leaves
- 0.9 oz (25 g) grated Parmesan cheese
- 2 cloves garlic, minced
- 1 tbsp lemon juice
- Salt and pepper to taste
- Red pepper flakes, for garnish (optional)

Directions:

1. In a food processor, combine the peeled avocados, olive oil, water, fresh basil leaves, fresh parsley leaves, grated Parmesan cheese, minced garlic, and lemon juice. Blend until smooth and creamy. If needed, add a bit more water to achieve the desired consistency. Season with salt and pepper to taste.
2. Heat a large skillet over medium heat. Add the halved cherry tomatoes and cook for about 2-3 minutes until they start to soften and release their juices. Remove the skillet from heat and set aside.
3. In the same skillet, add the spiralized zucchini noodles and cook for 2 minutes, just until they are heated through but still retain a slight crunch.
4. Pour the creamy avocado pesto over the zucchini noodles and toss to coat the noodles evenly.
5. Divide the creamy zucchini noodles among serving plates and top with the cooked cherry tomatoes.
6. If desired, sprinkle red pepper flakes over the dishes for an extra kick of heat.
7. Enjoy the dish.

Nutritional Values: Calories: 320 kcal | Fat: 25 g | Protein: 8 g | Carbs: 20 g | Net carbs: 14 g | Fiber: 6 g | Cholesterol: 5 mg | Sodium: 160 mg | Potassium: 1200 mg

Useful Tip: Feel free to customize the pesto by adding a handful of pine nuts or walnuts for added texture and flavor.

Mediterranean Stuffed Bell Peppers with Quinoa and Olives

Serving: 4 | Prep time: 20 minutes | Cook time: 35 minutes

Ingredients:

- 4 large bell peppers (assorted colors)
- 6 oz (180 g) quinoa, rinsed
- 16 oz (475 ml) vegetable broth
- 8 oz (225 g) canned chickpeas, drained and rinsed
- 2 oz (60 g) chopped Kalamata olives
- 1 oz (30 g) crumbled feta cheese
- 2 tbsp olive oil
- 1 small onion, finely chopped
- 2 cloves garlic, minced
- 1 tsp dried oregano
- 1 tsp dried basil
- Salt and pepper to taste
- Fresh parsley, chopped, for garnish

Directions:

1. Preheat the oven to 375°F (190°C).
2. Cut the tops off the bell peppers and remove the seeds and membranes. Place the peppers in a baking dish, cut side up.
3. In a saucepan, bring the vegetable broth to a boil. Add the rinsed quinoa, reduce the heat to low, cover, and let it simmer for about 15 minutes or until the quinoa is cooked and the liquid is absorbed. Fluff the quinoa with a fork.
4. In a large skillet, heat the olive oil over medium heat. Add the chopped onion and sauté for 2-3 minutes until it becomes translucent.
5. Stir in the minced garlic, dried oregano, and dried basil. Cook for another 1-2 minutes until fragrant.
6. Add the cooked quinoa, drained chickpeas, chopped Kalamata olives, and crumbled feta cheese to the skillet. Mix well to combine the ingredients.
7. Season the quinoa mixture with salt and pepper to taste.
8. Carefully stuff the bell peppers with the quinoa mixture, pressing down gently to pack it in.
9. Cover the baking dish with aluminum foil and bake in the preheated oven for 20 minutes.
10. Remove the foil and bake for an additional 5-10 minutes until the peppers are tender and slightly charred on top.
11. Garnish with chopped fresh parsley before serving.
12. Enjoy the dish.

Nutritional Values: Calories: 320 kcal | Fat: 10 g | Protein: 12 g | Carbs: 46 g | Net carbs: 34 g | Fiber: 12 g | Cholesterol: 10 mg | Sodium: 620 mg | Potassium: 970 mg

Useful Tip: Feel free to customize the stuffing by adding your favorite Mediterranean vegetables, such as diced tomatoes, artichoke hearts, or chopped spinach, for extra flavor and nutrition.

Cauliflower Rice Stir-Fry with Tofu and Ginger-Sesame Sauce

Serving: 4 | Prep time: 15 minutes | Cook time: 15 minutes
Ingredients:

- 16 oz (450 g) medium head of cauliflower, riced
- 14 oz (400 g) firm tofu, cubed
- 2 oz (30 ml) sesame oil
- 3 oz (45 ml) soy sauce (low-sodium)
- 1 oz (15 ml) rice vinegar
- 1 oz (15 ml) maple syrup or honey
- 0.35 oz (5 g) fresh ginger, grated

- 2 cloves garlic, minced
- 1 red bell pepper, sliced
- 4 oz (150 g) snap peas, trimmed and halved
- 2 green onions, sliced
- 0.35 oz (10 g) toasted sesame seeds
- 0.17 oz (5 ml) sriracha sauce (optional, for heat)

Directions:
1. Heat 1 ounce of sesame oil in a large skillet or wok over medium-high heat.
2. Add the cubed tofu and stir-fry until golden and slightly crispy, about 5-7 minutes. Remove tofu from the skillet and set aside.
3. In the same skillet, add the remaining ounce of sesame oil. Add the sliced red bell pepper and halved snap peas. Stir-fry for about 3-4 minutes until the vegetables are tender-crisp.
4. Push the vegetables to the side of the skillet and add the minced garlic and grated ginger to the center. Sauté for about 30 seconds until fragrant.
5. Combine the soy sauce, rice vinegar, maple syrup or honey, and sriracha sauce (if using) in a bowl to make the ginger-sesame sauce. Pour the sauce over the vegetables in the skillet and stir to coat.
6. Add the riced cauliflower to the skillet and stir-fry for another 3-4 minutes until the cauliflower is heated through and tender.
7. Return the cooked tofu to the skillet and toss everything together to combine.
8. Remove from heat and stir in the sliced green onions.
9. Serve the cauliflower rice stir-fry in bowls, garnished with toasted sesame seeds.
10. Enjoy the dish.

Nutritional Values: Calories: 280 kcal | Fat: 15 g | Protein: 18 g | Carbs: 22 g | Net carbs: 14 g | Fiber: 8 g | Cholesterol: 0 mg | Sodium: 580 mg | Potassium: 1050 mg
Useful Tip: For added flavor and crunch, sprinkle chopped roasted nuts, such as almonds or cashews, on top before serving.

Vegan Lentil Shepherd's Pie with Mashed Sweet Potato Topping

Serving: 4 | Prep time: 20 minutes | Cook time: 40 minutes
Ingredients:
For the Lentil Filling:

- 8 oz (225 g) brown lentils, cooked
- 1 oz (30 ml) olive oil
- 1 onion, chopped
- 2 carrots, diced
- 2 celery stalks, diced
- 2 cloves garlic, minced

- 1 tsp dried thyme
- 1 tsp paprika
- 8 oz (240 ml) vegetable broth
- 8 oz (240 ml) tomato sauce
- Salt and pepper to taste
- 4 oz (150 g) frozen peas

For the Mashed Sweet Potato Topping:

- 16 oz (450 g) large sweet potatoes, peeled and cubed
- 2 oz (60 ml) almond milk (unsweetened)

- 1 oz (30 ml) olive oil
- Salt and pepper to taste

Directions:
1. Preheat the oven to 375°F (190°C).
2. In a large skillet, heat the olive oil over medium heat. Add the chopped onion, diced carrots, and diced celery. Sauté for 5-6 minutes until the vegetables are tender.
3. Stir in the minced garlic, dried thyme, and paprika. Cook for an additional 1-2 minutes until fragrant.
4. Add the cooked lentils, vegetable broth, and tomato sauce to the skillet. Season with salt and pepper to taste. Simmer for 10-15 minutes until the mixture thickens.
5. Stir in the frozen peas and cook for another 2-3 minutes. Remove from heat.
6. Meanwhile, steam the cubed sweet potatoes until they are soft and tender, about 15-20 minutes. Drain and transfer to a mixing bowl.
7. Mash the sweet potatoes with almond milk, olive oil, salt, and pepper until smooth and creamy.
8. Transfer the lentil filling into a baking dish. Spread the mashed sweet potatoes evenly over the lentil mixture.
9. Bake in the preheated oven for 15-20 minutes, until the top is golden and the filling is bubbling.
10. Allow the pie to cool slightly before serving.
11. Enjoy the dish.

Nutritional Values: Calories: 320 kcal | Fat: 6 g | Protein: 14 g | Carbs: 54 g | Net carbs: 40 g | Fiber: 14 g | Cholesterol: 0 mg | Sodium: 620 mg | Potassium: 1350 mg
Useful Tip: Feel free to customize the mashed sweet potato topping by adding a pinch of cinnamon or nutmeg for extra warmth and flavor.

Roasted Butternut Squash and Black Bean Tacos with Cilantro-Lime Slaw

Serving: 4 | Prep time: 20 minutes | Cook time: 25 minutes

Ingredients: For the Roasted Butternut Squash:

- 16 oz (450 g) butternut squash, peeled, seeded, and cubed
- 2 oz (60 ml) olive oil
- 1 oz (5 g) ground cumin
- 1 oz (5 g) chili powder
- Salt and pepper to taste

For the Black Bean Filling:

- 15 oz (425 g) canned black beans, drained and rinsed
- 1 oz (30 ml) olive oil
- 1 oz (5 g) ground cumin
- 0.5 oz (2.5 g) smoked paprika
- Salt and pepper to taste

For the Cilantro-Lime Slaw:

- 4 oz (115 g) shredded cabbage or coleslaw mix
- 2 oz (60 ml) lime juice
- 2 oz (60 ml) olive oil
- 0.25 oz (15 g) chopped fresh cilantro
- Salt and pepper to taste

For Assembling:

- 8 small whole-grain or corn tortillas
- Sliced avocado, for garnish
- Lime wedges, for serving

Directions:

1. Preheat the oven to 400°F (200°C).
2. In a bowl, toss the cubed butternut squash with olive oil, ground cumin, chili powder, salt, and pepper. Spread evenly on a baking sheet and roast for about 20-25 minutes, until the squash is tender and slightly caramelized.
3. In a skillet, heat olive oil over medium heat. Add the drained black beans, ground cumin, smoked paprika, salt, and pepper. Cook for 3-4 minutes, stirring occasionally, until the beans are heated through and well-coated with the spices. Remove from heat.
4. In a separate bowl, whisk together lime juice, olive oil, chopped cilantro, salt, and pepper. Toss the shredded cabbage or coleslaw mix with the cilantro-lime dressing to make the slaw.
5. Warm the tortillas in a dry skillet over medium heat for about 30 seconds on each side.
6. To assemble the tacos, spoon the roasted butternut squash and black bean filling onto each tortilla. Top with a generous amount of cilantro-lime slaw and sliced avocado.
7. Serve the tacos with lime wedges on the side.
8. Enjoy the dish.

Nutritional Values: Calories: 320 kcal | Fat: 12 g | Protein: 10 g | Carbs: 47 g | Net carbs: 32 g | Fiber: 15 g | Cholesterol: 0 mg | Sodium: 460 mg | Potassium: 930 mg

Useful Tip: For added protein, you can include a dollop of non-dairy yogurt or sprinkle with pumpkin seeds on top of the tacos before serving.

Creamy Mushroom and Spinach Pasta with Cashew Alfredo Sauce

Serving: 4 | Prep time: 15 minutes | Cook time: 20 minutes

Ingredients:

- 12 oz (340 g) whole wheat pasta
- 8 oz (225 g) button mushrooms, sliced
- 4 oz (115 g) baby spinach
- 1 oz (30 ml) olive oil

- 2 cloves garlic, minced
- 1 tsp dried thyme
- Salt and pepper to taste

For the Cashew Alfredo Sauce:

- 4 oz (115 g) raw cashews, soaked and drained
- 8 oz (240 ml) unsweetened almond milk
- 2 tbsp nutritional yeast

- 1 tbsp lemon juice
- 2 cloves garlic
- Salt and pepper to taste

Directions:

1. Cook the whole wheat pasta according to the package instructions. Drain and set aside.
2. In a large skillet, heat the olive oil over medium heat. Add the sliced mushrooms and sauté for 5-6 minutes until they are golden brown and tender.
3. Stir in the minced garlic and dried thyme. Cook for another minute until fragrant.
4. Add the baby spinach to the skillet and cook until wilted. Season with salt and pepper to taste.
5. For the Cashew Alfredo Sauce, blend the soaked cashews, almond milk, nutritional yeast, lemon juice, and cloves of garlic in a blender until smooth and creamy. Season with salt and pepper to taste.
6. Combine the cooked pasta, sautéed mushrooms and spinach, and the Cashew Alfredo Sauce in the skillet. Mix well to coat the pasta and vegetables with the sauce.
7. Heat the pasta over low heat for a few minutes to warm everything through.
8. Serve the creamy mushroom and spinach pasta in bowls.
9. Enjoy the dish.

Nutritional Values: Calories: 420 kcal | Fat: 16 g | Protein: 16 g | Carbs: 58 g | Net carbs: 48 g | Fiber: 10 g | Cholesterol: 0 mg | Sodium: 340 mg | Potassium: 750 mg

Useful Tip: For extra protein, you can add cooked chickpeas or white beans to the dish for a heartier meal.

Spaghetti Squash Pad Thai with Peanut Sauce and Tofu

Serving: 4 | Prep time: 20 minutes | Cook time: 30 minutes

Ingredients:

- 1 medium spaghetti squash (about 3 lbs / 1350 g)
- 8 oz (225 g) firm tofu, cubed
- 2 oz (60 ml) olive oil
- 2 cloves garlic, minced

- 2 oz (60 g) bean sprouts

- 2 carrots, julienned
- 1 red bell pepper, julienned
- 2 green onions, sliced

- 2 oz (60 g) chopped roasted peanuts

For the Peanut Sauce:

- 4 oz (115 g) natural peanut butter
- 2 oz (60 ml) soy sauce (low-sodium)
- 1 oz (30 ml) lime juice
- 1 oz (30 ml) rice vinegar
- 1 oz (30 ml) water

- 1 tbsp maple syrup or honey
- 1 tsp minced ginger
- 1 clove garlic, minced
- 0.5 oz (15 g) chopped cilantro (for garnish)
- Lime wedges, for serving

Directions:

1. Preheat the oven to 375°F (190°C).
2. Cut the spaghetti squash in half lengthwise and scoop out the seeds. Place the halves cut side down on a baking sheet and roast for about 25-30 minutes, until the flesh can be easily scraped into spaghetti-like strands with a fork.
3. In a skillet, heat 1 ounce of olive oil over medium heat. Add the cubed tofu and cook until golden and slightly crispy. Remove from the skillet and set aside.

4. In the same skillet, add the remaining ounce of olive oil. Sauté the minced garlic until fragrant.
5. Add the julienned carrots and red bell pepper to the skillet and stir-fry for about 2-3 minutes until the vegetables are slightly tender.
6. Add the cooked spaghetti squash strands, cooked tofu, sliced green onions, and bean sprouts to the skillet. Toss everything together.
7. In a bowl, whisk together the peanut butter, soy sauce, lime juice, rice vinegar, water, maple syrup or honey, minced ginger, and minced garlic to make the peanut sauce.
8. Pour the peanut sauce over the spaghetti squash mixture in the skillet. Toss well to coat everything with the sauce.
9. Serve the Spaghetti Squash Pad Thai in bowls, garnished with chopped roasted peanuts and cilantro. Serve with lime wedges on the side.
10. Enjoy the dish.

Nutritional Values: Calories: 420 kcal | Fat: 28 g | Protein: 14 g | Carbs: 35 g | Net carbs: 25 g | Fiber: 10 g | Cholesterol: 0 mg | Sodium: 530 mg | Potassium: 860 mg

Useful Tip: Feel free to customize the dish with additional vegetables such as snow peas, broccoli, or edamame for added flavor and nutrition.

Vegan Black Bean Chili with Cornbread Muffins

Serving: 4 | Prep time: 15 minutes | Cook time: 30 minutes
Ingredients:

For the Black Bean Chili:

- 16 oz (450 g) canned black beans, drained and rinsed
- 8 oz (225 g) diced tomatoes (canned or fresh)
- 4 oz (115 g) diced bell peppers (assorted colors)
- 4 oz (115 g) diced onions
- 2 cloves garlic, minced
- 1 oz (30 ml) olive oil

- 1 oz (5 g) chili powder
- 1 tsp ground cumin
- 1 tsp paprika
- 0.5 tsp cayenne pepper (adjust to taste)
- Salt and pepper to taste
- 8 oz (240 ml) vegetable broth

For the Cornbread Muffins:

- 8 oz (225 g) cornmeal
- 4 oz (115 g) whole wheat flour
- 1 oz (30 g) coconut sugar or other sweetener
- 2 tsp baking powder

- 0.5 tsp salt
- 8 oz (240 ml) unsweetened almond milk
- 2 oz (60 ml) apple cider vinegar
- 2 oz (60 ml) olive oil

Directions:
1. In a large pot, heat the olive oil over medium heat. Add the diced onions, bell peppers, and minced garlic. Sauté for 3-4 minutes until the vegetables are slightly softened.
2. Stir in the chili powder, ground cumin, paprika, cayenne pepper, salt, and pepper. Cook for an additional 2 minutes until the spices are fragrant.
3. Add the diced tomatoes, drained black beans, and vegetable broth to the pot. Bring to a simmer and let the chili cook for about 15-20 minutes, allowing the flavors to meld.
4. While the chili is simmering, preheat the oven to 400°F (200°C) and line a muffin tin with paper liners.
5. In a bowl, whisk together the cornmeal, whole wheat flour, coconut sugar, baking powder, and salt for the cornbread muffins.
6. In a separate bowl, mix together the almond milk, apple cider vinegar, and olive oil. Add the wet ingredients to the dry ingredients and stir until just combined.
7. Divide the cornbread batter evenly among the muffin cups and bake for about 15-18 minutes, or until a toothpick inserted into the center comes out clean.
8. Serve the Vegan Black Bean Chili topped with desired toppings alongside the freshly baked Cornbread Muffins.
9. Enjoy the dish.

Nutritional Values: Calories: 450 kcal | Fat: 16 g | Protein: 12 g | Carbs: 70 g | Net carbs: 50 g | Fiber: 20 g | Cholesterol: 0 mg | Sodium: 600 mg | Potassium: 750 mg

Useful Tip: Garnish your chili with chopped fresh cilantro, avocado slices, or a dollop of dairy-free yogurt for added flavor and creaminess.

Moroccan Chickpea and Vegetable Tagine with Apricots and Almonds

Serving: 4 | Prep time: 20 minutes | Cook time: 40 minutes

Ingredients:

- 16 oz (450 g) canned chickpeas, drained and rinsed
- 8 oz (225 g) diced tomatoes (canned or fresh)
- 4 oz (115 g) diced carrots
- 4 oz (115 g) diced bell peppers (assorted colors)
- 4 oz (115 g) diced zucchini
- 2 oz (60 g) diced onions
- 2 cloves garlic, minced
- 1 oz (30 ml) olive oil
- 2 oz (60 g) dried apricots, chopped
- 2 oz (60 g) slivered almonds
- 1 oz (30 g) tomato paste
- 2 tsp ground cumin
- 1 tsp ground coriander
- 1 tsp ground paprika
- 0.5 tsp ground cinnamon
- 0.25 tsp ground turmeric
- 16 oz (480 ml) vegetable broth
- Salt and pepper to taste
- Fresh cilantro, for garnish

Directions:

1. In a large tagine or skillet, heat the olive oil over medium heat. Add the diced onions and sauté for 3-4 minutes until they start to soften.
2. Stir in the minced garlic, ground cumin, ground coriander, ground paprika, ground cinnamon, and ground turmeric. Cook for an additional 2 minutes until the spices are fragrant.
3. Add the diced carrots, bell peppers, and zucchini to the tagine. Sauté for about 5 minutes until the vegetables begin to soften.
4. Stir in the tomato paste and diced tomatoes. Cook for another 3-4 minutes to allow the flavors to meld.
5. Add the canned chickpeas and dried apricots to the tagine. Pour in the vegetable broth, season with salt and pepper, and give everything a good stir.
6. Cover the tagine and let the mixture simmer for 20-25 minutes, allowing the flavors to develop and the vegetables to become tender.
7. While the tagine is simmering, toast the slivered almonds in a dry skillet over medium heat until they are golden and fragrant. Set aside.
8. Once the tagine is ready, serve it in bowls, garnished with the toasted slivered almonds and fresh cilantro.
9. Enjoy the dish.

Nutritional Values: Calories: 380 kcal | Fat: 14 g | Protein: 12 g | Carbs: 55 g | Net carbs: 40 g | Fiber: 15 g | Cholesterol: 0 mg | Sodium: 800 mg | Potassium: 980 mg

Useful Tip: Serve the Moroccan Chickpea and Vegetable Tagine over cooked quinoa or whole wheat couscous for a complete and satisfying meal.

Roasted Brussels Sprouts and Quinoa Salad with Balsamic Glaze

Serving: 4 | Prep time: 15 minutes | Cook time: 25 minutes

Ingredients:

For the Salad:

- 12 oz (340 g) Brussels sprouts, trimmed and halved
- 4 oz (115 g) quinoa, rinsed and drained
- 2 oz (60 g) chopped pecans
- 2 oz (60 g) dried cranberries
- 2 oz (60 g) chopped red onion
- 1 oz (30 ml) olive oil
- Salt and pepper to taste

For the Balsamic Glaze:

- 2 oz (60 ml) balsamic vinegar
- 1 oz (30 ml) olive oil
- 1 tsp Dijon mustard
- 1 tsp honey or maple syrup (optional)
- Salt and pepper to taste

Directions:

1. Preheat the oven to 400°F (200°C).
2. Toss the halved Brussels sprouts with olive oil, salt, and pepper. Spread them on a baking sheet and roast for about 20-25 minutes, until they are tender and slightly crispy on the edges.

3. While the Brussels sprouts are roasting, cook the quinoa according to package instructions. Once cooked, fluff with a fork and let it cool slightly.
4. In a small bowl, whisk together the balsamic vinegar, olive oil, Dijon mustard, honey or maple syrup (if using), salt, and pepper to make the balsamic glaze.
5. In a large bowl, combine the roasted Brussels sprouts, cooked quinoa, chopped pecans, dried cranberries, and chopped red onion.
6. Drizzle the balsamic glaze over the salad and toss everything together until well coated.
7. Serve the Roasted Brussels Sprouts and Quinoa Salad in bowls, garnished with extra pecans if desired.
8. Enjoy the dish.

Nutritional Values: Calories: 350 kcal | Fat: 18 g | Protein: 8 g | Carbs: 40 g | Net carbs: 30 g | Fiber: 6 g | Cholesterol: 0 mg | Sodium: 80 mg | Potassium: 480 mg

Useful Tip: For an extra burst of flavor, add crumbled feta cheese or goat cheese to the salad before drizzling with the balsamic glaze.

Vegan Spinach and Artichoke Stuffed Portobello Mushrooms

Serving: 4 | Prep time: 20 minutes | Cook time: 25 minutes

Ingredients:

- 4 large Portobello mushrooms
- 8 oz (225 g) fresh spinach
- 4 oz (115 g) canned artichoke hearts, drained and chopped
- 2 oz (60 g) diced onion
- 2 cloves garlic, minced
- 2 oz (60 g) vegan cream cheese
- 2 oz (60 g) vegan mozzarella cheese, shredded
- 1 oz (30 ml) olive oil
- Salt and pepper to taste
- Fresh chopped parsley, for garnish

Directions:

1. Preheat the oven to 375°F (190°C).
2. Remove the stems from the Portobello mushrooms and gently scrape out the gills with a spoon. Place the mushrooms on a baking sheet.
3. In a skillet, heat the olive oil over medium heat. Add the diced onion and minced garlic. Sauté for 2-3 minutes until the onion is translucent.
4. Add the fresh spinach to the skillet and cook until wilted. Remove from heat and let cool slightly.
5. In a bowl, combine the cooked spinach, chopped artichoke hearts, vegan cream cheese, and half of the shredded vegan mozzarella cheese. Mix well and season with salt and pepper.
6. Divide the spinach and artichoke mixture evenly among the Portobello mushrooms, stuffing each mushroom cap.
7. Top the stuffed mushrooms with the remaining shredded vegan mozzarella cheese.
8. Bake in the preheated oven for about 20-25 minutes, until the mushrooms are tender and the cheese is melted and bubbly.
9. Garnish the Vegan Spinach and Artichoke Stuffed Portobello Mushrooms with fresh chopped parsley before serving.
10. Enjoy the dish.

Nutritional Values: Calories: 240 kcal | Fat: 15 g | Protein: 8 g | Carbs: 19 g | Net carbs: 14 g | Fiber: 5 g | Cholesterol: 0 mg | Sodium: 480 mg | Potassium: 810 mg

Useful Tip: Feel free to customize the stuffing by adding chopped sun-dried tomatoes, roasted red peppers, or chopped nuts for added texture and flavor.

Sweet Potato and Chickpea Curry with Coconut Milk and Curry Leaves

Serving: 4 | Prep time: 15 minutes | Cook time: 25 minutes

Ingredients:

- 16 oz (450 g) sweet potatoes, peeled and diced
- 12 oz (340 g) canned chickpeas, drained and rinsed
- 8 oz (225 g) diced tomatoes (canned or fresh)
- 4 oz (115 g) diced onions
- 2 oz (60 g) chopped bell peppers (assorted colors)
- 2 oz (60 g) chopped carrots
- 1 oz (30 g) coconut oil
- 1 oz (30 ml) olive oil
- 14 oz (400 ml) canned coconut milk
- 1 oz (30 g) tomato paste
- 10-12 fresh curry leaves
- 1 tsp ground turmeric
- 1 tsp ground cumin
- 1 tsp ground coriander
- 0.5 tsp red chili flakes (adjust to taste)
- Salt and pepper to taste
- Fresh cilantro, for garnish

Directions:

1. In a large skillet or pot, heat the coconut oil over medium heat. Add the diced onions and sauté for 3-4 minutes until they start to soften.
2. Stir in the ground turmeric, ground cumin, ground coriander, and red chili flakes. Cook for an additional 2 minutes until the spices are fragrant.
3. Add the diced sweet potatoes, chopped bell peppers, and chopped carrots to the skillet. Sauté for about 5 minutes until the vegetables begin to soften.
4. Stir in the tomato paste, diced tomatoes, and fresh curry leaves. Cook for another 3-4 minutes to allow the flavors to meld.
5. Pour in the canned coconut milk and season with salt and pepper. Bring the mixture to a simmer and cook for 10-12 minutes, until the sweet potatoes are tender.
6. Add the canned chickpeas to the curry and cook for an additional 5 minutes to heat them through.
7. Drizzle with olive oil and garnish with fresh cilantro before serving.
8. Enjoy the dish.

Nutritional Values: Calories: 380 kcal | Fat: 20 g | Protein: 8 g | Carbs: 42 g | Net carbs: 34 g | Fiber: 8 g | Cholesterol: 0 mg | Sodium: 380 mg | Potassium: 970 mg

Useful Tip: Serve the Sweet Potato and Chickpea Curry with steamed brown rice or quinoa for a well-balanced and satisfying meal.

Lentil and Vegetable Stir-Fry with Quinoa and Ginger-Sesame Sauce

Serving: 4 | Prep time: 15 minutes | Cook time: 20 minutes

Ingredients:

- 8 oz (225 g) cooked quinoa
- 8 oz (225 g) cooked green or brown lentils
- 6 oz (170 g) sliced bell peppers (assorted colors)
- 4 oz (115 g) sliced carrots
- 4 oz (115 g) broccoli florets
- 2 oz (60 g) diced onions
- 2 oz (60 g) snow peas, trimmed
- 1 oz (30 ml) sesame oil
- 1 oz (30 ml) low-sodium soy sauce
- 1 oz (30 ml) rice vinegar
- 1 oz (30 ml) water
- 1 oz (30 g) natural peanut butter
- 1 tsp minced ginger
- 1 tsp minced garlic
- 0.5 tsp red pepper flakes (adjust to taste)
- 1 tbsp maple syrup or agave nectar
- 1 oz (28 g) chopped peanuts, for garnish
- Fresh cilantro, for garnish

Directions:

1. In a large wok or skillet, heat the sesame oil over medium-high heat. Add the diced onions and sauté for 2-3 minutes until they start to soften.
2. Add the sliced bell peppers, sliced carrots, and broccoli florets to the wok. Stir-fry for about 5-7 minutes until the vegetables are tender-crisp.
3. In a bowl, whisk together the low-sodium soy sauce, rice vinegar, water, peanut butter, minced ginger, minced garlic, red pepper flakes, and maple syrup.
4. Pour the sauce over the stir-fried vegetables and add the cooked quinoa and lentils. Toss everything together to coat well and heat through.
5. Add the trimmed snow peas to the wok and cook for an additional 2 minutes until they are vibrant and slightly tender.
6. Divide the lentil and vegetable stir-fry among serving plates.
7. Garnish with chopped peanuts and fresh cilantro.
8. Enjoy the dish.

Nutritional Values: Calories: 350 kcal | Fat: 12 g | Protein: 15 g | Carbs: 45 g | Net carbs: 33 g | Fiber: 12 g | Cholesterol: 0 mg | Sodium: 550 mg | Potassium: 750 mg

Useful Tip: Feel free to customize the vegetables in this stir-fry based on your preferences and what's in season.

Roasted Beet and Orange Salad with Arugula and Maple-Mustard Dressing

Serving: 4 | Prep time: 15 minutes | Cook time: 30 minutes
Ingredients:

- 16 oz (450 g) beets, peeled and diced
- 4 oz (115 g) baby arugula
- 2 oranges, peeled and segmented
- 1 oz (30 g) chopped walnuts
- 1 oz (30 g) crumbled goat cheese (optional)
- 1 oz (30 ml) olive oil
- 1 oz (30 ml) balsamic vinegar
- 1 tbsp maple syrup
- 1 tsp Dijon mustard
- Salt and pepper to taste

Directions:
1. Preheat the oven to 400°F (200°C).
2. Place the diced beets on a baking sheet and drizzle with olive oil. Season with salt and pepper and toss to coat evenly. Roast the beets in the preheated oven for about 25-30 minutes, or until they are tender and slightly caramelized.
3. In a small bowl, whisk together the balsamic vinegar, maple syrup, Dijon mustard, and a pinch of salt and pepper to make the dressing.
4. In a large salad bowl, arrange the baby arugula, roasted beets, orange segments, chopped walnuts, and crumbled goat cheese (if using).
5. Drizzle the maple-mustard dressing over the salad and toss gently to combine.
6. Divide the salad among serving plates.
7. Enjoy the dish.

Nutritional Values: Calories: 220 kcal | Fat: 14 g | Protein: 4 g | Carbs: 20 g | Net carbs: 16 g | Fiber: 4 g | Cholesterol: 5 mg | Sodium: 220 mg | Potassium: 480 mg
Useful Tip: To save time, you can roast the beets in advance and store them in the refrigerator until ready to use in the salad.

Vegan Mediterranean Pizza with Cauliflower Crust and Hummus Spread

Serving: 4 | Prep time: 20 minutes | Cook time: 25 minutes
Ingredients:
For the Cauliflower Crust:

- 16 oz (450 g) cauliflower florets
- 2 oz (60 g) almond flour
- 1 oz (30 g) nutritional yeast
- 1 tsp garlic powder
- 1 tsp dried oregano
- Salt and pepper to taste
- 1 fl oz (30 ml) olive oil

For the Hummus Spread:

- 8 oz (225 g) canned chickpeas, drained and rinsed
- 2 oz (60 ml) tahini
- 2 oz (60 ml) lemon juice
- 1 garlic clove
- Salt and pepper to taste

Toppings:

- 4 oz (115 g) cherry tomatoes, halved
- 2 oz (60 g) Kalamata olives, pitted and sliced
- 2 oz (60 g) red onion, thinly sliced
- 2 oz (60 g) baby spinach
- 1 oz (30 g) chopped fresh parsley
- 1 oz (30 ml) extra virgin olive oil

Directions:
1. Preheat the oven to 425°F (220°C).
2. In a food processor, pulse the cauliflower florets until they resemble fine crumbs.
3. Transfer the cauliflower crumbs to a clean kitchen towel and squeeze out excess moisture.
4. In a bowl, combine the cauliflower crumbs, almond flour, nutritional yeast, garlic powder, dried oregano, salt, and pepper.
5. Form the cauliflower mixture into a ball and place it on a parchment-lined baking sheet. Flatten and shape it into a round crust, about ¼ inch thick.
6. Bake the crust in the preheated oven for 15-20 minutes, until it's golden and firm.
7. While the crust is baking, prepare the hummus spread by blending the chickpeas, tahini, lemon juice, garlic clove, salt, and pepper in a food processor until smooth.
8. Once the crust is ready, spread the hummus over the surface.
9. Arrange the cherry tomatoes, Kalamata olives, red onion, and baby spinach on top of the hummus.
10. Drizzle with extra virgin olive oil and sprinkle chopped fresh parsley over the pizza.
11. Return the pizza to the oven and bake for an additional 5-7 minutes until the toppings are heated through.
12. Slice the pizza and serve.

Nutritional Values: Calories: 320 kcal | Fat: 22 g | Protein: 10 g | Carbs: 25 g | Net carbs: 18 g | Fiber: 7 g | Cholesterol: 0 mg | Sodium: 350 mg | Potassium: 750 mg
Useful Tip: For added flavor, you can sprinkle some crushed red pepper flakes over the pizza before baking or serving if you prefer a spicier kick. Enjoy the pizza with a side salad for a complete meal.

Grilled Eggplant and Zucchini Roll-Ups with Sun-Dried Tomato Pesto

Serving: 4 | Prep time: 20 minutes | Cook time: 15 minutes

Ingredients:

For the Roll-Ups:

- 1 medium eggplant, sliced lengthwise into thin strips
- 2 medium zucchinis, sliced lengthwise into thin strips
- 2 oz (60 ml) olive oil
- Salt and pepper to taste

For the Sun-Dried Tomato Pesto:

- 2 oz (60 g) sun-dried tomatoes (not packed in oil), soaked in hot water and drained
- 1 oz (30 g) almonds
- 1 oz (30 ml) olive oil
- 1 garlic clove
- 1 oz (30 g) fresh basil leaves
- Juice of 1 lemon
- Salt and pepper to taste

For Assembly:

- 2 oz (60 g) baby spinach leaves
- 2 oz (60 g) vegan cheese shreds (optional)

Directions:

1. Preheat a grill or grill pan over medium heat.
2. Brush the eggplant and zucchini slices with olive oil and season with salt and pepper.
3. Grill the eggplant and zucchini slices for about 2-3 minutes on each side until they have grill marks and are tender. Remove from heat and set aside.
4. In a food processor, combine the soaked sun-dried tomatoes, almonds, olive oil, garlic clove, fresh basil leaves, lemon juice, salt, and pepper. Process until a smooth pesto forms.
5. Lay out the grilled eggplant and zucchini slices on a clean surface.
6. Spread a thin layer of the sun-dried tomato pesto onto each slice.
7. Place a few baby spinach leaves on top of the pesto.
8. If using, sprinkle vegan cheese shreds over the spinach.
9. Gently roll up the slices to create the roll-ups.
10. Serve the roll-ups as an appetizer, snack, or light meal.

Nutritional Values: Calories: 180 kcal | Fat: 12 g | Protein: 5 g | Carbs: 15 g | Net carbs: 10 g | Fiber: 5 g | Cholesterol: 0 mg | Sodium: 240 mg | Potassium: 800 mg

Useful Tip: To make the roll-ups easier to handle, secure each roll-up with a toothpick before serving. These roll-ups can also be served as a colorful and flavorful appetizer at parties or gatherings. Enjoy the dish with a side salad for a well-rounded meal.

Mediterranean Chickpea and Quinoa Bowl with Lemon-Herb Vinaigrette

Serving: 4 | Prep time: 15 minutes | Cook time: 20 minutes

Ingredients:

For the Bowl:

- 8 oz (225 g) cooked quinoa
- 16 oz (450 g) canned chickpeas, drained and rinsed
- 6 oz (170 g) cherry tomatoes, halved
- 4 oz (115 g) cucumber, diced
- 2 oz (60 g) red onion, finely chopped
- 2 oz (60 g) Kalamata olives, pitted and sliced
- 2 oz (60 g) crumbled feta cheese (optional)
- 1 oz (30 g) chopped fresh parsley
- 1 oz (30 g) chopped fresh mint
- Salt and pepper to taste

For the Lemon-Herb Vinaigrette:

- 2 oz (60 ml) extra-virgin olive oil
- 1 oz (30 ml) fresh lemon juice
- 1 garlic clove, minced
- 1 tsp Dijon mustard
- 1 tsp honey or maple syrup
- 1 tsp dried oregano
- Salt and pepper to taste

Directions:

1. In a large bowl, combine the cooked quinoa, chickpeas, cherry tomatoes, cucumber, red onion, Kalamata olives, and crumbled feta cheese (if using).
2. In a separate small bowl, whisk together the extra-virgin olive oil, fresh lemon juice, minced garlic, Dijon mustard, honey or maple syrup, dried oregano, salt, and pepper to create the vinaigrette.

3. Pour the Lemon-Herb Vinaigrette over the quinoa and chickpea mixture and toss to combine.
4. Add chopped fresh parsley and mint to the bowl and gently toss again to distribute the herbs.
5. Season the bowl with additional salt and pepper if needed.
6. Divide the Mediterranean chickpea and quinoa mixture into serving bowls.
7. Enjoy the dish with a refreshing and tangy flavor of the lemon-herb vinaigrette.

Nutritional Values: Calories: 320 kcal | Fat: 16 g | Protein: 10 g | Carbs: 35 g | Net carbs: 30 g | Fiber: 5 g | Cholesterol: 5 mg | Sodium: 400 mg | Potassium: 550 mg

Useful Tip: Feel free to customize this Mediterranean Chickpea and Quinoa Bowl with your favorite veggies, such as bell peppers, artichoke hearts, or roasted red peppers. The lemon-herb vinaigrette can be prepared in advance and stored in the refrigerator for up to a week to use in various salads and bowls. Enjoy the dish as a wholesome and satisfying meal or as a light lunch option.

Cucumber and Hummus Stuffed Mini Bell Peppers

Serving: 4 | Prep time: 15 minutes | Cook time: 0 minutes
Ingredients:

- 16 mini bell peppers
- 8 oz (225 g) cucumber, finely diced
- 8 oz (225 g) prepared hummus
- 2 oz (60 g) diced red onion
- 2 oz (60 g) diced cherry tomatoes
- 2 oz (60 g) diced Kalamata olives
- 2 oz (60 g) crumbled feta cheese (optional)
- 1 oz (30 g) chopped fresh parsley
- 1 oz (30 g) chopped fresh dill
- 1 oz (30 ml) extra-virgin olive oil
- 1 oz (30 ml) balsamic vinegar
- Salt and pepper to taste

Directions:
1. Carefully slice off the tops of the mini bell peppers and remove the seeds and membranes.
2. In a mixing bowl, combine the finely diced cucumber, diced red onion, diced cherry tomatoes, and diced Kalamata olives.
3. Add the chopped fresh parsley and dill to the bowl and mix well.
4. In a separate small bowl, whisk together the extra-virgin olive oil, balsamic vinegar, salt, and pepper to create a simple dressing.
5. Pour the dressing over the cucumber and veggie mixture and toss to coat the ingredients evenly.
6. Fill each mini bell pepper with a spoonful of prepared hummus.
7. Stuff each bell pepper with the cucumber and veggie mixture, pressing gently to pack it in.
8. Optionally, sprinkle crumbled feta cheese over the stuffed peppers for added flavor.
9. Arrange the stuffed mini bell peppers on a serving platter.
10. Enjoy the dish as a delightful appetizer or snack.

Nutritional Values: Calories: 180 kcal | Fat: 10 g | Protein: 5 g | Carbs: 18 g | Net carbs: 15 g | Fiber: 3 g | Cholesterol: 5 mg | Sodium: 380 mg | Potassium: 350 mg

Useful Tip: For a dairy-free option, omit the crumbled feta cheese. You can also use flavored hummus varieties to add different tastes to your stuffed mini bell peppers. These stuffed peppers can be prepared in advance and stored in the refrigerator for a quick and nutritious snack or appetizer option. Enjoy the dish as a colorful and flavorful addition to your meals.

Crunchy Kale Chips with Nutritional Yeast and Garlic Powder

Serving: 4 | Prep time: 10 minutes | Cook time: 20 minutes
Ingredients:

- 10 oz (280 g) kale leaves, stems removed and torn into bite-sized pieces
- 1 oz (30 ml) olive oil
- 1 oz (30 g) nutritional yeast
- 1 tsp garlic powder
- Salt to taste

Directions:
1. Preheat the oven to 300°F (150°C).
2. In a large bowl, combine the torn kale leaves with olive oil and toss until well coated.
3. Spread the kale pieces in a single layer on a baking sheet lined with parchment paper.
4. Sprinkle nutritional yeast, garlic powder, and a pinch of salt evenly over the kale leaves.
5. Bake in the preheated oven for 15-20 minutes, or until the kale chips are crisp and edges are lightly browned.
6. Remove from the oven and allow the kale chips to cool slightly before serving.
7. Transfer the kale chips to a serving bowl and enjoy them as a crunchy and flavorful snack.

Nutritional Values: Calories: 100 kcal | Fat: 5 g | Protein: 6 g | Carbs: 10 g | Net carbs: 5 g | Fiber: 5 g | Cholesterol: 0 mg | Sodium: 140 mg | Potassium: 700 mg

Useful Tip: Ensure that the kale leaves are thoroughly dry before tossing them with olive oil. You can use a salad spinner or pat them dry with a kitchen towel. Experiment with different seasonings like chili powder, smoked paprika, or lemon zest for alternative flavors. Store leftover kale chips in an airtight container to maintain their crispiness. Enjoy this nutritious and satisfying snack as a guilt-free alternative to traditional chips.

Zucchini Fritters with Lemon-Herb Greek Yogurt Dip

Serving: 4 | Prep time: 20 minutes | Cook time: 15 minutes
Ingredients:

For Zucchini Fritters:
- 16 oz (450 g) zucchini, grated and squeezed to remove excess moisture
- 4 oz (115 g) onion, finely chopped
- 2 cloves garlic, minced
- 4 oz (115 g) almond flour
- 2 oz (60 g) grated Parmesan cheese (optional)
- 2 oz (60 g) chopped fresh parsley
- 2 oz (60 g) chopped fresh dill
- 1 oz (30 g) chopped green onions
- 2 large eggs
- Salt and pepper to taste
- 2 oz (60 ml) olive oil, for frying

For Lemon-Herb Greek Yogurt Dip:
- 8 oz (225 g) Greek yogurt
- 1 oz (30 ml) fresh lemon juice
- 1 tsp lemon zest
- 1 oz (30 g) chopped fresh mint
- 1 oz (30 g) chopped fresh dill
- Salt and pepper to taste

Directions:
1. In a large bowl, combine the grated zucchini, chopped onion, minced garlic, almond flour, grated Parmesan cheese (if using), chopped parsley, chopped dill, chopped green onions, eggs, salt, and pepper. Mix until well combined.
2. Heat olive oil in a skillet over medium heat.
3. Using a spoon, scoop portions of the zucchini mixture and gently flatten them into patties. Place the patties in the skillet and cook for about 3-4 minutes on each side, or until golden brown and crispy. Cook in batches if needed.
4. Remove the fritters from the skillet and place them on a paper towel-lined plate to remove any excess oil.
5. For Lemon-Herb Greek Yogurt Dip: In a small bowl, combine Greek yogurt, fresh lemon juice, lemon zest, chopped mint, chopped dill, salt, and pepper. Mix well.
6. To Serve: Arrange the zucchini fritters on a serving platter.
7. Serve with the Lemon-Herb Greek Yogurt Dip on the side.
8. Enjoy the dish as a tasty and nutritious appetizer or snack.

Nutritional Values: Calories: 260 kcal | Fat: 18 g | Protein: 12 g | Carbs: 14 g | Net carbs: 9 g | Fiber: 5 g | Cholesterol: 85 mg | Sodium: 350 mg | Potassium: 750 mg

Useful Tip: To achieve crispy fritters, make sure to squeeze out as much moisture from the grated zucchini as possible before mixing the ingredients. The Lemon-Herb Greek Yogurt Dip adds a refreshing tangy flavor to the fritters and can be used as a dip for various dishes. Experiment with different herbs and spices to personalize the flavors of your fritters and dip.

Baked Sweet Potato Fries with Cumin and Paprika

Serving: 4 | Prep time: 15 minutes | Cook time: 25 minutes
Ingredients:

- 32 oz (900 g) sweet potatoes, peeled and cut into fries
- 2 oz (60 ml) olive oil
- 1 tsp ground cumin
- 1 tsp paprika
- Salt and pepper to taste
- Fresh parsley or cilantro, chopped (for garnish)

Directions:
1. Preheat the oven to 425°F (220°C).
2. In a large bowl, toss the sweet potato fries with olive oil, ground cumin, paprika, salt, and pepper until well coated.
3. Arrange the coated sweet potato fries in a single layer on a baking sheet lined with parchment paper.
4. Bake in the preheated oven for about 20-25 minutes, flipping the fries halfway through, until they are golden and crispy.
5. Remove the fries from the oven and transfer them to a serving platter.
6. Garnish with chopped fresh parsley or cilantro.
7. Serve the baked sweet potato fries as a delicious and healthier alternative to traditional fries.

Nutritional Values: Calories: 220 kcal | Fat: 7 g | Protein: 3 g | Carbs: 38 g | Net carbs: 32 g | Fiber: 6 g | Cholesterol: 0 mg | Sodium: 230 mg | Potassium: 700 mg

Useful Tip: For extra crispiness, make sure to spread out the sweet potato fries in a single layer on the baking sheet without overcrowding. You can customize the seasoning by adding your favorite herbs and spices to enhance the flavor of the fries. Serve the baked sweet potato fries with a healthy dipping sauce such as Greek yogurt mixed with lemon juice and fresh herbs. Enjoy the dish as a satisfying and guilt-free snack or side dish.

Coconut-Covered Date and Nut Energy Balls

Serving: 4 | Prep time: 15 minutes | Cook time: 0 minutes

Ingredients:

- 8 oz (225 g) pitted dates
- 4 oz (115 g) mixed nuts (such as almonds, walnuts, and cashews)
- 2 oz (60 g) unsweetened shredded coconut, plus extra for rolling
- 1 oz (30 ml) coconut oil, melted
- 1 tsp vanilla extract
- 0.5 tsp ground cinnamon
- Pinch of salt

Directions:

1. In a food processor, combine the pitted dates, mixed nuts, shredded coconut, melted coconut oil, vanilla extract, ground cinnamon, and a pinch of salt.
2. Process the mixture until it forms a sticky and cohesive dough.
3. Take small portions of the dough and roll them into bite-sized balls using your hands.
4. Spread some extra shredded coconut on a plate.
5. Roll each energy ball in the shredded coconut, pressing gently to coat them evenly.
6. Place the coated energy balls on a parchment-lined tray.
7. Refrigerate the energy balls for at least 30 minutes to firm up.
8. Once firm, transfer the energy balls to an airtight container and store in the refrigerator.

Nutritional Values: Calories: 140 kcal | Fat: 8 g | Protein: 2 g | Carbs: 15 g | Net carbs: 13 g | Fiber: 2 g | Cholesterol: 0 mg | Sodium: 5 mg | Potassium: 210 mg

Useful Tip: Feel free to customize these energy balls by adding your favorite mix-ins, such as chopped dried fruits, chocolate chips, or seeds. If the mixture is too sticky to handle, wet your hands with a little water to make the rolling process easier. These energy balls are a great on-the-go snack or a healthy dessert alternative when you need a quick burst of energy. Enjoy the dish as a tasty and nutritious treat that satisfies your cravings while providing natural sweetness and healthy fats.

Spicy Edamame and Sesame Snack Mix

Serving: 4 | Prep time: 10 minutes | Cook time: 15 minutes

Ingredients:

- 8 oz (225 g) frozen edamame, thawed
- 4 oz (115 g) unsalted mixed nuts (almonds, cashews, walnuts)
- 2 oz (60 g) pumpkin seeds
- 1 oz (30 g) sesame seeds
- 1 oz (30 ml) low-sodium soy sauce
- 1 oz (30 ml) toasted sesame oil
- 1 tsp sriracha sauce (adjust to taste)
- 0.5 tsp garlic powder
- 0.5 tsp onion powder
- 0.25 tsp cayenne pepper (adjust to taste)
- Salt to taste

Directions:

1. Preheat the oven to 350°F (175°C).
2. In a bowl, combine the thawed edamame, mixed nuts, pumpkin seeds, and sesame seeds.
3. In a separate bowl, whisk together the low-sodium soy sauce, toasted sesame oil, sriracha sauce, garlic powder, onion powder, cayenne pepper, and a pinch of salt.
4. Pour the sauce mixture over the nut and seed mixture and toss until everything is well coated.
5. Spread the mixture evenly on a baking sheet lined with parchment paper.
6. Bake in the preheated oven for about 12-15 minutes, stirring occasionally, until the nuts and seeds are toasted and golden brown.
7. Remove from the oven and let the snack mix cool completely before serving.

Nutritional Values: Calories: 180 kcal | Fat: 14 g | Protein: 10 g | Carbs: 7 g | Net carbs: 5 g | Fiber: 2 g | Cholesterol: 0 mg | Sodium: 300 mg | Potassium: 240 mg

Useful Tip: Feel free to adjust the level of spiciness to your taste preferences by increasing or decreasing the amount of sriracha and cayenne pepper. This snack mix is a satisfying and flavorful option for when you're craving something crunchy and spicy. Store the snack mix in an airtight container to keep it fresh for longer periods. Enjoy the dish as a protein-packed snack that's perfect for satisfying your hunger and giving you an energy boost between meals.

Mashed Avocado and Tomato Bruschetta on Whole Wheat Crackers

Serving: 4 | Prep time: 10 minutes | Cook time: 0 minutes

Ingredients:

- 2 ripe avocados
- 1 large tomato, diced
- 2 cloves garlic, minced
- 2 tbsp fresh lemon juice
- 2 tbsp extra-virgin olive oil

- 0.5 tsp red pepper flakes (adjust to taste)
- Salt and pepper to taste
- 16 whole wheat crackers
- Fresh basil leaves, for garnish

Directions:

1. In a mixing bowl, scoop out the flesh of the ripe avocados and mash them with a fork until smooth.
2. Stir in the diced tomato, minced garlic, fresh lemon juice, and extra-virgin olive oil.
3. Add red pepper flakes, salt, and pepper, and mix well to combine all the flavors.
4. Taste and adjust the seasoning if needed.
5. Spoon the mashed avocado and tomato mixture onto each whole wheat cracker.
6. Garnish with fresh basil leaves.
7. Serve immediately and enjoy this delicious and nutritious snack!

Nutritional Values: Calories: 180 kcal | Fat: 14 g | Protein: 3 g | Carbs: 13 g | Net carbs: 9 g | Fiber: 4 g | Cholesterol: 0 mg | Sodium: 150 mg | Potassium: 400 mg

Useful Tip: To prevent the mashed avocado from browning, you can press a piece of plastic wrap directly onto the surface of the mixture before refrigerating. This simple and flavorful bruschetta recipe is a great option for a light and satisfying snack or appetizer. The healthy fats from the avocado, combined with the fresh tomato and basil, provide a burst of flavor that pairs perfectly with the whole wheat crackers. Enjoy this dish as a nutrient-rich addition to your GOLO Diet meal plan!

Smoked Salmon Cucumber Bites with Dill Cream Cheese

Serving: 4 | Prep time: 15 minutes | Cook time: 0 minutes

Ingredients:

- 1 large cucumber
- 4 oz (115 g) smoked salmon, thinly sliced
- 4 oz (115 g) cream cheese, softened

- 1 tbsp fresh lemon juice
- 2 tbsp fresh dill, chopped
- Salt and pepper to taste

Directions:

1. Wash and peel the cucumber, leaving some strips of skin for visual appeal.
2. Slice the cucumber into rounds, about 1/4 inch thick.
3. In a bowl, mix the softened cream cheese, fresh lemon juice, chopped dill, salt, and pepper until well combined.
4. Spread a small amount of the dill cream cheese mixture onto each cucumber round.
5. Place a slice of smoked salmon on top of the cream cheese layer.
6. Garnish with additional dill if desired.
7. Arrange the smoked salmon cucumber bites on a serving platter.
8. Serve immediately and enjoy this elegant and nutritious appetizer!

Nutritional Values: Calories: 120 kcal | Fat: 8 g | Protein: 8 g | Carbs: 3 g | Net carbs: 2 g | Fiber: 1 g | Cholesterol: 30 mg | Sodium: 300 mg | Potassium: 170 mg

Useful Tip: To make the cream cheese easier to spread, allow it to come to room temperature before mixing. These smoked salmon cucumber bites make a delightful and low-carb option for gatherings or as a light snack. The combination of the cool cucumber, creamy dill-infused cream cheese, and savory smoked salmon creates a burst of flavors and textures that's sure to satisfy your taste buds while keeping you on track with your GOLO Diet. Enjoy this recipe as a delicious way to enjoy the benefits of nutrient-rich ingredients!

Spicy Tuna Lettuce Wraps with Avocado and Sriracha Mayo

Serving: 4 | Prep time: 20 minutes | Cook time: 0 minutes

Ingredients:

- 12 oz (340 g) canned tuna in water, drained
- 2 large avocados, peeled, pitted, and diced
- 2 oz (60 ml) mayonnaise
- 1 oz (30 ml) sriracha sauce (adjust to taste)
- 2 oz (60 ml) fresh lemon juice
- 0.4 oz (10 g) fresh cilantro, chopped
- Salt and pepper to taste
- 8 large lettuce leaves (such as butter lettuce or iceberg)

Directions:

1. In a bowl, combine the drained canned tuna, diced avocado, chopped cilantro, and fresh lemon juice.
2. In a separate bowl, mix the mayonnaise and sriracha sauce to create the spicy mayo.
3. Gently fold the spicy mayo into the tuna and avocado mixture until well combined.
4. Season with salt and pepper to taste.
5. Place a scoop of the spicy tuna and avocado mixture onto each lettuce leaf.
6. Roll up the lettuce leaves to create wraps, securing them with toothpicks if needed.
7. Arrange the lettuce wraps on a serving platter.
8. Serve immediately, and enjoy the bold flavors and satisfying crunch of these Spicy Tuna Lettuce Wraps!

Nutritional Values: Calories: 250 kcal | Fat: 18 g | Protein: 14 g | Carbs: 8 g | Net carbs: 4 g | Fiber: 4 g | Cholesterol: 25 mg | Sodium: 300 mg | Potassium: 650 mg

Useful Tip: Adjust the level of spiciness by adding more or less sriracha sauce to the mayo mixture, depending on your preference. These Spicy Tuna Lettuce Wraps are not only delicious but also a great source of protein, healthy fats, and fiber. They make a fantastic light meal or snack option that fits well with the GOLO Diet principles. Enjoy the convenience of this recipe and the burst of flavors it brings to your taste buds!

Baked Mini Meatballs with Roasted Cherry Tomatoes

Serving: 4 | Prep time: 15 minutes | Cook time: 20 minutes

Ingredients:

- 16 oz (450 g) ground lean turkey or chicken
- 1 oz (30 g) grated Parmesan cheese
- 1 oz (30 g) whole wheat bread crumbs
- 1 oz (30 g) diced onion
- 1 oz (30 g) chopped fresh parsley
- 1 oz (30 ml) milk
- 1 oz (30 ml) olive oil
- 2 oz (60 g) egg whites (approximately 2 large egg whites)
- 1 oz (30 g) chopped garlic
- Salt and pepper to taste
- 16 oz (450 g) cherry tomatoes
- 0.5 oz (15 ml) balsamic vinegar

Directions:

1. Preheat the oven to 400°F (200°C).
2. In a bowl, combine the ground lean turkey or chicken, grated Parmesan cheese, whole wheat bread crumbs, diced onion, chopped fresh parsley, milk, olive oil, egg whites, chopped garlic, salt, and pepper.
3. Mix the ingredients until well combined.
4. Shape the mixture into mini meatballs, approximately 1 inch in diameter.
5. Place the meatballs on a baking sheet lined with parchment paper.
6. In a separate bowl, toss the cherry tomatoes with balsamic vinegar.
7. Arrange the balsamic-coated cherry tomatoes around the meatballs on the baking sheet.
8. Bake in the preheated oven for about 20 minutes, or until the meatballs are cooked through and the cherry tomatoes are roasted and slightly caramelized.
9. Serve the baked mini meatballs with the roasted cherry tomatoes as a flavorful and protein-rich meal.

Nutritional Values: Calories: 280 kcal | Fat: 14 g | Protein: 25 g | Carbs: 15 g | Net carbs: 11 g | Fiber: 4 g | Cholesterol: 70 mg | Sodium: 380 mg | Potassium: 680 mg

Useful Tip: For a variation, consider using lean ground beef, ground pork, or a combination of different ground meats. You can also customize the seasoning of the meatballs with herbs and spices of your choice, following the GOLO Diet guidelines. These baked mini meatballs with roasted cherry tomatoes can be served over a bed of cooked whole grains or with a side of steamed vegetables for a well-balanced meal. Enjoy the convenience and rich flavors of this recipe as part of your GOLO Diet journey!

Berry Blast Frozen Yogurt Popsicles with Granola Crunch

Serving: 4 | Prep time: 10 minutes | Freeze time: 4 hours
Ingredients:

- 6 oz (170 g) mixed berries (such as strawberries, blueberries, raspberries)
- 8 oz (225 g) plain Greek yogurt
- 1 oz (30 ml) honey or maple syrup
- 1 oz (30 g) granola
- 0.5 oz (15 ml) lemon juice
- 0.5 oz (15 ml) water
- 1 oz (30 ml) unsweetened almond milk or milk of choice

Directions:

1. In a blender or food processor, combine the mixed berries, Greek yogurt, honey or maple syrup, lemon juice, and water.
2. Blend until you have a smooth berry-yogurt mixture.
3. In a separate bowl, mix the granola with almond milk or milk of your choice until it's slightly softened.
4. Gently fold the granola mixture into the berry-yogurt mixture to create a crunchy texture.
5. Carefully pour the mixture into popsicle molds, leaving a little space at the top to allow for expansion as they freeze.
6. Insert popsicle sticks into the molds and place them in the freezer.
7. Freeze the popsicles for at least 4 hours, or until they are completely frozen.
8. To remove the popsicles from the molds, run the molds briefly under warm water to help release them.
9. Enjoy these delicious Berry Blast Frozen Yogurt Popsicles with Granola Crunch as a refreshing and satisfying treat!

Nutritional Values: Calories: 110 kcal | Fat: 2 g | Protein: 6 g | Carbs: 18 g | Net carbs: 14 g | Fiber: 4 g | Cholesterol: 0 mg | Sodium: 35 mg | Potassium: 160 mg

Useful Tip: Feel free to customize these popsicles by using different types of berries or adding a sprinkle of cinnamon or a dash of vanilla extract to the berry-yogurt mixture for extra flavor. Be mindful of portion sizes to stay within the guidelines of the GOLO Diet. These popsicles can be a satisfying and guilt-free dessert option that includes the goodness of yogurt and antioxidant-rich berries. Enjoy them during warmer months or whenever you're in the mood for a cool and tasty treat!

Almond Flour Chocolate Chip Cookies with Coconut and Walnuts

Serving: 4 | Prep time: 15 minutes | Cook time: 12 minutes
Ingredients:

- 6 oz (170 g) almond flour
- 2 oz (60 g) unsweetened shredded coconut
- 2 oz (60 g) chopped walnuts
- 2 oz (60 g) dark chocolate chips (at least 70% cocoa)
- 1 oz (30 ml) coconut oil, melted
- 1 oz (30 ml) honey or maple syrup
- 1 tsp vanilla extract
- 1 egg
- 0.5 tsp baking soda
- Pinch of salt

Directions:

1. Preheat the oven to 350°F (175°C) and line a baking sheet with parchment paper.
2. In a large bowl, mix together the almond flour, shredded coconut, chopped walnuts, dark chocolate chips, baking soda, and a pinch of salt.
3. In a separate bowl, whisk together the melted coconut oil, honey or maple syrup, vanilla extract, and egg until well combined.
4. Pour the wet ingredients into the dry ingredients and mix until a dough forms.
5. Using a spoon or cookie scoop, drop spoonfuls of dough onto the prepared baking sheet, spacing them a few inches apart.
6. Gently flatten each cookie with the back of a spoon to create a cookie shape.
7. Bake in the preheated oven for about 10-12 minutes, or until the edges are golden brown.
8. Remove the cookies from the oven and allow them to cool on the baking sheet for a few minutes before transferring them to a wire rack to cool completely.
9. Once the cookies are completely cool, enjoy these delicious Almond Flour Chocolate Chip Cookies with Coconut and Walnuts as a satisfying and healthier dessert option.

Nutritional Values: Calories: 180 kcal | Fat: 15 g | Protein: 5 g | Carbs: 10 g | Net carbs: 6 g | Fiber: 4 g | Cholesterol: 20 mg | Sodium: 70 mg | Potassium: 150 mg

Useful Tip: To keep these cookies soft and chewy, store them in an airtight container with a piece of bread or a slice of apple to maintain moisture. The natural oils in almond flour and coconut oil can make the cookies more delicate, so handle them gently when transferring to the cooling rack. These cookies are a great treat for those following the GOLO Diet, providing a balance of healthy fats and satisfying flavors without excessive refined sugars. Enjoy them as a guilt-free dessert or snack option!

Roasted Peach and Ricotta Parfait with Honey Drizzle

Serving: 4 | Prep time: 15 minutes | Cook time: 15 minutes

Ingredients:

- 4 ripe peaches, pitted and sliced
- 2 oz (60 g) ricotta cheese
- 1 oz (30 ml) honey
- 1 oz (30 g) chopped walnuts
- 1 oz (30 g) granola
- 1 tsp coconut oil
- 1/2 tsp vanilla extract
- Pinch of cinnamon

Directions:

1. Preheat the oven to 375°F (190°C).
2. In a bowl, toss the peach slices with the coconut oil and a pinch of cinnamon until evenly coated.
3. Spread the peach slices on a baking sheet lined with parchment paper and roast in the preheated oven for about 15 minutes, until the peaches are tender and slightly caramelized.
4. In a separate bowl, mix the ricotta cheese with vanilla extract until smooth.
5. In serving glasses or bowls, layer the roasted peach slices, a dollop of ricotta cheese, a sprinkle of chopped walnuts, and a layer of granola.
6. Repeat the layers until the glasses are filled.
7. Drizzle honey over the top of each parfait.
8. Serve immediately or refrigerate until ready to enjoy.

Nutritional Values: Calories: 150 kcal | Fat: 7 g | Protein: 4 g | Carbs: 20 g | Net carbs: 16 g | Fiber: 4 g | Cholesterol: 10 mg | Sodium: 20 mg | Potassium: 220 mg

Useful Tip: Choose ripe peaches for maximum flavor and sweetness. You can customize this parfait by using different types of nuts, such as almonds or pecans, and swapping the ricotta for Greek yogurt if desired. Be mindful of portion sizes, as the natural sugars in fruits can add up. This Roasted Peach and Ricotta Parfait with Honey Drizzle is a delightful way to enjoy a balanced and satisfying dessert that includes fiber, protein, and healthy fats, making it a great option for those following the GOLO Diet. Enjoy it as a light and flavorful treat after a meal!

Cinnamon-Spiced Baked Apples with Pecan Streusel

Serving: 4 | Prep time: 15 minutes | Cook time: 25 minutes

Ingredients:

- 4 medium apples (such as Granny Smith or Honeycrisp)
- 2 oz (60 g) chopped pecans
- 1 oz (30 g) almond flour
- 1 oz (30 g) coconut sugar
- 1 oz (30 ml) melted coconut oil
- 1 tsp ground cinnamon
- 1/2 tsp vanilla extract
- Pinch of salt

Directions:

1. Preheat the oven to 375°F (190°C).
2. Core the apples and carefully scoop out some of the flesh to create a well for the filling. Leave about 1/2 inch of apple around the edges.
3. In a bowl, combine the chopped pecans, almond flour, coconut sugar, melted coconut oil, ground cinnamon, vanilla extract, and a pinch of salt. Mix until the streusel topping is well combined.
4. Fill each cored apple with the pecan streusel mixture, pressing it down gently.
5. Place the filled apples in a baking dish and bake in the preheated oven for about 25 minutes, or until the apples are tender and the streusel is golden brown.
6. Remove from the oven and let the baked apples cool slightly before serving.

Nutritional Values: Calories: 220 kcal | Fat: 17 g | Protein: 2 g | Carbs: 17 g | Net carbs: 12 g | Fiber: 5 g | Cholesterol: 0 mg | Sodium: 20 mg | Potassium: 180 mg

Useful Tip: Select apples that are firm and have a sweet-tart flavor for the best results in this recipe. You can adjust the sweetness by using more or less coconut sugar according to your taste preferences. Enjoy these Cinnamon-Spiced Baked Apples with Pecan Streusel as a healthier dessert option that's rich in fiber, healthy fats, and natural sweetness. Serve them warm with a dollop of Greek yogurt or a drizzle of almond butter for extra flavor and creaminess. These baked apples make for a comforting and satisfying treat that's perfect for a cozy evening. Enjoy the dish!

Lemon Blueberry Chia Seed Pudding with Toasted Almonds

Serving: 4 | Prep time: 10 minutes | Cook time: 0 minutes

Ingredients:

- 2 oz (56 g) chia seeds
- 16 oz (480 ml) unsweetened almond milk
- Zest and juice of 1 lemon
- 1 oz (28 g) blueberries
- 1 oz (28 g) toasted almonds, chopped
- 1 tbsp pure maple syrup (optional, for sweetness)
- 1/2 tsp vanilla extract

Directions:

1. In a mixing bowl, combine the chia seeds, unsweetened almond milk, lemon zest, lemon juice, vanilla extract, and pure maple syrup (if using). Stir well to ensure the chia seeds are evenly distributed.
2. Let the mixture sit for about 10-15 minutes, stirring occasionally, until it thickens to a pudding-like consistency.
3. Gently fold in the blueberries, reserving a few for garnish.
4. Divide the chia seed pudding mixture into serving glasses or jars.
5. Top each serving with chopped toasted almonds and the reserved blueberries.
6. Refrigerate the chia seed pudding for at least 1-2 hours, or until fully chilled and set.
7. Before serving, give the pudding a quick stir to evenly distribute the ingredients.
8. Enjoy the Lemon Blueberry Chia Seed Pudding with Toasted Almonds as a nutritious and delicious breakfast or snack option.

Nutritional Values: Calories: 150 kcal | Fat: 9 g | Protein: 5 g | Carbs: 15 g | Net carbs: 9 g | Fiber: 6 g | Cholesterol: 0 mg | Sodium: 120 mg | Potassium: 180 mg

Useful Tip: Toasting the almonds before adding them to the pudding enhances their flavor and adds a satisfying crunch. You can customize the sweetness of the pudding by adjusting the amount of maple syrup according to your preference. Experiment with different berries, such as raspberries or strawberries, for variety. This Lemon Blueberry Chia Seed Pudding with Toasted Almonds is a great make-ahead option, and you can prepare it the night before to have a hassle-free breakfast or snack ready to enjoy.

Dark Chocolate-Dipped Banana Bites with Sea Salt

Serving: 4 | Prep time: 15 minutes | Cook time: 5 minutes

Ingredients:

- 2 large bananas, ripe but firm
- 4 oz (115 g) dark chocolate (70% cocoa or higher), chopped
- 1 tsp coconut oil
- Pinch of sea salt
- 1 oz (28 g) chopped nuts (such as almonds, walnuts, or pistachios), for garnish

Directions:

1. Line a baking sheet with parchment paper.
2. Peel the bananas and cut them into bite-sized slices, about 1/2-inch thick.
3. In a microwave-safe bowl or using a double boiler, melt the dark chocolate and coconut oil together until smooth.
4. Dip each banana slice halfway into the melted chocolate, then place it on the prepared baking sheet.
5. While the chocolate is still wet, sprinkle a pinch of sea salt over each chocolate-dipped banana slice.
6. Optional: Sprinkle chopped nuts over the chocolate-dipped side of the banana slices for added crunch.
7. Place the baking sheet in the refrigerator for about 10-15 minutes, or until the chocolate hardens.
8. Once the chocolate is set, transfer the banana bites to a serving platter.
9. Enjoy the Dark Chocolate-Dipped Banana Bites with Sea Salt as a delectable treat or dessert.

Nutritional Values: Calories: 120 kcal | Fat: 6 g | Protein: 2 g | Carbs: 16 g | Net carbs: 12 g | Fiber: 4 g | Cholesterol: 0 mg | Sodium: 20 mg | Potassium: 250 mg

Useful Tip: Ensure the bananas are ripe but still slightly firm for the best texture when dipping in chocolate. Experiment with different types of dark chocolate, adjusting the cocoa percentage to suit your taste preferences. Adding a pinch of sea salt not only enhances the flavors but also balances the sweetness of the chocolate and bananas. If you're looking to add an extra layer of flavor, try sprinkling a touch of ground cinnamon or crushed red pepper flakes over the chocolate-dipped banana bites before they set. This treat is best enjoyed immediately or kept in the refrigerator for a refreshing and indulgent snack.

Mini Pumpkin Spice Energy Bites with Cranberries and Almonds

Serving: 4 | Prep time: 15 minutes | Cook time: 0 minutes

Ingredients:

- 6 oz (170 g) pitted dates
- 1.75 oz (50 g) rolled oats
- 1.75 oz (50 g) almond flour
- 1 oz (30 g) dried cranberries
- 1 oz (30 g) chopped almonds
- 2 tbsp pumpkin puree
- 1 tsp pure maple syrup
- 1/2 tsp pumpkin spice blend
- 1/2 tsp vanilla extract
- Pinch of salt
- Unsweetened shredded coconut, for rolling (optional)

Directions:

1. In a food processor, combine pitted dates, rolled oats, almond flour, dried cranberries, chopped almonds, pumpkin puree, maple syrup, pumpkin spice blend, vanilla extract, and a pinch of salt.
2. Pulse the mixture until it comes together and forms a sticky dough.
3. Using your hands, roll the dough into bite-sized balls, about 1 inch in diameter.
4. Optional: Roll the energy bites in unsweetened shredded coconut to coat the exterior.
5. Place the energy bites on a parchment-lined tray and refrigerate for about 30 minutes to firm up.
6. Once chilled, transfer the energy bites to an airtight container and store in the refrigerator for up to a week.
7. Enjoy the Mini Pumpkin Spice Energy Bites with Cranberries and Almonds as a quick and nutritious snack.

Nutritional Values: Calories: 120 kcal | Fat: 5 g | Protein: 2 g | Carbs: 18 g | Net carbs: 15 g | Fiber: 3 g | Cholesterol: 0 mg | Sodium: 10 mg | Potassium: 180 mg

Useful Tip: If you prefer a sweeter taste, you can adjust the amount of maple syrup to suit your taste preferences. These energy bites can be customized by adding other ingredients like chia seeds, flax seeds, or even a sprinkle of cinnamon. Keep in mind that almond flour adds a nutty flavor and contributes to the overall texture of the energy bites. You can store these energy bites in the freezer for longer-term storage, making them a convenient and satisfying snack option whenever you need a boost of energy. Enjoy these bites as a pre-workout snack, a mid-afternoon pick-me-up, or a guilt-free dessert.

Vanilla Coconut Rice Pudding with Fresh Mango Slices

Serving: 4 | Prep time: 10 minutes | Cook time: 30 minutes

Ingredients:

- 3.5 oz (100 g) Arborio rice
- 13.5 oz (400 ml) light coconut milk
- 10 oz (280 ml) unsweetened almond milk
- 2 oz (60 g) granulated sugar or sweetener of choice
- 1 vanilla bean or 1 tsp vanilla extract
- Pinch of salt
- 1 fresh mango, peeled and sliced
- Unsweetened shredded coconut, for garnish (optional)

Directions:

1. In a medium-sized saucepan, combine Arborio rice, light coconut milk, almond milk, granulated sugar, and a pinch of salt.
2. If using a vanilla bean, split it open and scrape out the seeds. Add the seeds and the vanilla bean pod (or vanilla extract) to the saucepan.
3. Bring the mixture to a gentle simmer over medium heat, stirring occasionally to prevent sticking.
4. Reduce the heat to low and continue to cook the rice pudding, stirring occasionally, for about 25-30 minutes or until the rice is tender and the mixture has thickened.
5. Remove the vanilla bean pod if used, and discard it.
6. Let the rice pudding cool slightly before dividing it into serving bowls.
7. Top each bowl with fresh mango slices and a sprinkle of unsweetened shredded coconut, if desired.
8. Serve the Vanilla Coconut Rice Pudding with Fresh Mango Slices warm or chilled.

Nutritional Values: Calories: 200 kcal | Fat: 7 g | Protein: 2 g | Carbs: 32 g | Net carbs: 27 g | Fiber: 5 g | Cholesterol: 0 mg | Sodium: 40 mg | Potassium: 250 mg

Useful Tip: Feel free to adjust the sweetness of the rice pudding by using more or less sugar/sweetener according to your taste preferences. The rice pudding will thicken further as it cools, so if you prefer a thinner consistency, you can add a little more almond milk while cooking. For added texture and flavor, you can stir in toasted sliced almonds or chopped nuts. This comforting dessert can be enjoyed as a satisfying and indulgent treat while still staying within the guidelines of the Golo Diet. Enjoy the creamy richness of the rice pudding paired with the natural sweetness of fresh mango slices for a delightful combination of flavors and textures.

Raspberry Almond Flour Muffins with Lemon Glaze

Serving: 4 | Prep time: 15 minutes | Cook time: 20 minutes

Ingredients:

- 7 oz (200 g) almond flour
- 1.5 oz (45 g) coconut flour
- 2 tsp baking powder
- 3.5 oz (100 g) raspberries
- 3.5 oz (100 g) unsalted butter, melted and cooled
- 3.5 oz (100 g) granulated sweetener of choice
- 3 large eggs
- 2 tsp vanilla extract
- Zest of 1 lemon
- Pinch of salt

For the Lemon Glaze:

- 1 oz (30 g) powdered sweetener of choice
- Juice of 1 lemon

Directions:

1. Preheat the oven to 350°F (175°C) and line a muffin tin with paper liners.
2. In a bowl, whisk together the almond flour, coconut flour, baking powder, and a pinch of salt.
3. In a separate bowl, beat the eggs and granulated sweetener until well combined and slightly frothy.
4. Add the melted butter, vanilla extract, and lemon zest to the egg mixture and mix well.
5. Gradually add the dry ingredients to the wet ingredients and mix until a smooth batter forms.
6. Gently fold in the raspberries.
7. Divide the batter evenly among the muffin cups, filling each about 2/3 full.
8. Bake in the preheated oven for 18-20 minutes, or until a toothpick inserted into the center of a muffin comes out clean.
9. While the muffins are baking, prepare the lemon glaze by whisking together the powdered sweetener and lemon juice until smooth.
10. Once the muffins are done, remove them from the oven and let them cool for a few minutes before transferring them to a wire rack to cool completely.
11. Drizzle the lemon glaze over the cooled muffins.
12. Allow the glaze to set before serving.

Nutritional Values: Calories: 210 kcal | Fat: 18 g | Protein: 6 g | Carbs: 8 g | Net carbs: 4 g | Fiber: 4 g | Cholesterol: 105 mg | Sodium: 300 mg | Potassium: 160 mg

Useful Tip: To avoid making the muffins too sweet, choose a granulated sweetener that is compatible with the Golo Diet. Feel free to use fresh or frozen raspberries, and consider folding some raspberries into the batter while reserving a few to place on top before baking for a burst of flavor in every bite. The lemon glaze adds a tangy and zesty touch, enhancing the overall taste of these delightful muffins. Enjoy these Raspberry Almond Flour Muffins with Lemon Glaze as a delicious breakfast or snack option that fits well within the guidelines of the Golo Diet.

Spiced Carrot Cake Oat Bars with Cream Cheese Drizzle

Serving: 4 | Prep time: 15 minutes | Cook time: 25 minutes

Ingredients:

- 5.3 oz (150 g) rolled oats
- 2 oz (60 g) almond flour
- 1 tsp baking powder
- 1 tsp ground cinnamon
- 1/2 tsp ground nutmeg
- 1/4 tsp ground ginger
- Pinch of salt
- 2 large carrots, grated
- 2 oz (60 g) unsweetened applesauce
- 2 oz (60 g) Greek yogurt
- 2 oz (60 g) granulated sweetener of choice
- 1 large egg
- 1 tsp vanilla extract

For the Cream Cheese Drizzle:

- 2 oz (60 g) cream cheese, softened
- 1 oz (30 g) powdered sweetener of choice
- 1 tsp vanilla extract

Directions:

1. Preheat the oven to 350°F (175°C) and line a baking dish with parchment paper.
2. In a bowl, combine the rolled oats, almond flour, baking powder, ground cinnamon, nutmeg, ginger, and a pinch of salt.
3. In a separate bowl, whisk together the grated carrots, applesauce, Greek yogurt, granulated sweetener, egg, and vanilla extract.

4. Gradually add the dry ingredients to the wet ingredients and mix until well combined.
5. Pour the batter into the prepared baking dish and spread it evenly.
6. Bake in the preheated oven for 20-25 minutes, or until the edges are golden brown and a toothpick inserted into the center comes out clean.
7. While the bars are baking, prepare the cream cheese drizzle by mixing together the softened cream cheese, powdered sweetener, and vanilla extract until smooth.
8. Once the bars are done baking, let them cool slightly before drizzling the cream cheese mixture over the top.
9. Allow the bars to cool completely before slicing into squares.

Nutritional Values: Calories: 220 kcal | Fat: 10 g | Protein: 6 g | Carbs: 25 g | Net carbs: 17 g | Fiber: 8 g | Cholesterol: 45 mg | Sodium: 180 mg | Potassium: 280 mg

Useful Tip: To keep the bars moist and flavorful, make sure to grate the carrots finely to evenly distribute their natural sweetness throughout the batter. The combination of warm spices, almond flour, and Greek yogurt adds both flavor and texture to these oat bars, making them a delightful treat that aligns with the principles of the Golo Diet. Enjoy these Spiced Carrot Cake Oat Bars with Cream Cheese Drizzle as a satisfying snack or dessert option that's rich in fiber and protein.

Chocolate Avocado Mousse with Berries and Cocoa Nibs

Serving: 4 | Prep time: 10 minutes | Cook time: 0 minutes

Ingredients:

- 2 ripe avocados, pitted and peeled
- 3 oz (85 g) dark chocolate, melted and cooled
- 2 oz (60 g) unsweetened cocoa powder
- 2 oz (60 g) powdered sweetener of choice
- 1 tsp vanilla extract
- Pinch of salt
- 4 oz (115 g) mixed berries (such as strawberries, blueberries, raspberries)
- 1 oz (30 g) cocoa nibs

Directions:

1. In a food processor, combine the ripe avocados, melted dark chocolate, unsweetened cocoa powder, powdered sweetener, vanilla extract, and a pinch of salt.
2. Blend the ingredients until smooth and creamy, scraping down the sides of the food processor as needed.
3. Divide the chocolate avocado mousse into 4 serving glasses or bowls.
4. Top each serving with a variety of mixed berries and a sprinkle of cocoa nibs.
5. Chill the mousse in the refrigerator for at least 30 minutes before serving.

Nutritional Values: Calories: 220 kcal | Fat: 15 g | Protein: 4 g | Carbs: 20 g | Net carbs: 12 g | Fiber: 8 g | Cholesterol: 0 mg | Sodium: 5 mg | Potassium: 500 mg

Useful Tip: When selecting avocados for this recipe, choose ripe ones with a slightly soft texture. This will ensure that the avocado blends smoothly into the mousse, creating a creamy and luscious texture. The addition of mixed berries and cocoa nibs provides a burst of flavor and crunch to complement the rich chocolate avocado mousse, making it a satisfying and guilt-free dessert option that adheres to the Golo Diet principles. Enjoy the delightful combination of flavors and textures in this Chocolate Avocado Mousse with Berries and Cocoa Nibs.

Baked Pear Halves with Cinnamon and Greek Yogurt

Serving: 4 | Prep time: 10 minutes | Cook time: 25 minutes

Ingredients:

- 2 ripe pears, halved and cored
- 1 oz (30 g) chopped walnuts
- 1 tsp ground cinnamon
- 2 tbsp honey or maple syrup
- 6 oz (170 g) plain Greek yogurt

Directions:

1. Preheat the oven to 350°F (175°C).
2. Place the pear halves on a baking sheet, cut side up.
3. In a small bowl, mix the chopped walnuts with ground cinnamon.
4. Sprinkle the cinnamon-walnut mixture evenly over the pear halves.
5. Drizzle honey or maple syrup over the pears.
6. Bake the pears in the preheated oven for about 25 minutes, or until they are tender and the tops are slightly caramelized.
7. Allow the baked pear halves to cool slightly before serving.
8. Serve each pear half with a dollop of plain Greek yogurt.

Nutritional Values: Calories: 150 kcal | Fat: 5 g | Protein: 6 g | Carbs: 25 g | Net carbs: 20 g | Fiber: 5 g | Cholesterol: 0 mg | Sodium: 15 mg | Potassium: 300 mg

Useful Tip: Choose pears that are ripe but still firm for this recipe. Baking them will soften them further, and they'll become tender and flavorful with a hint of caramelization. Greek yogurt provides a creamy and tangy contrast to the sweetness of the baked pears, making this a satisfying and balanced dessert option that aligns with the Golo Diet principles. Enjoy the warm and comforting flavors of Baked Pear Halves with Cinnamon and Greek Yogurt, perfect for a healthy and indulgent treat.

Mini Chocolate Protein Pancakes with Raspberry Sauce

Serving: 4 | Prep time: 15 minutes | Cook time: 15 minutes

Ingredients:

- 4 oz (115 g) chocolate protein powder
- 2 oz (55 g) almond flour
- 1 tsp baking powder
- 1/2 tsp ground cinnamon
- 2 large eggs
- 4 oz (120 ml) unsweetened almond milk
- 1 oz (30 g) dark chocolate chips
- 1 cup fresh raspberries
- 1 tbsp honey or maple syrup
- Cooking spray

Directions:

1. In a bowl, whisk together the chocolate protein powder, almond flour, baking powder, and ground cinnamon.
2. In a separate bowl, beat the eggs and mix in the unsweetened almond milk.
3. Gradually add the wet ingredients to the dry ingredients and mix until smooth. Fold in the dark chocolate chips.
4. Heat a non-stick skillet over medium heat. Lightly grease with cooking spray.
5. Pour small spoonfuls of batter onto the skillet to form mini pancakes. Cook for about 2 minutes on each side or until lightly browned.
6. In a blender, combine the fresh raspberries and honey or maple syrup. Blend until smooth to make the raspberry sauce.
7. Serve the mini chocolate protein pancakes with a drizzle of raspberry sauce on top.

Nutritional Values: Calories: 220 kcal | Fat: 9 g | Protein: 20 g | Carbs: 15 g | Net carbs: 10 g | Fiber: 5 g | Cholesterol: 85 mg | Sodium: 180 mg | Potassium: 250 mg

Useful Tip: For the best consistency in your mini pancakes, make sure to blend the wet and dry ingredients thoroughly. These mini chocolate protein pancakes are a delicious and nutritious breakfast option that provides a good balance of protein and fiber to keep you satisfied and energized. The raspberry sauce adds a burst of fruity flavor without added sugars, making this recipe a great choice for a satisfying morning meal. Enjoy the delightful combination of flavors in Mini Chocolate Protein Pancakes with Raspberry Sauce, and start your day with a nutritious treat.

Chia Seed Coconut Macaroons with Dark Chocolate Drizzle

Serving: 4 | Prep time: 10 minutes | Cook time: 20 minutes

Ingredients:

- 2 oz (60 g) chia seeds
- 4 oz (115 g) unsweetened shredded coconut
- 2 oz (60 ml) coconut milk
- 1 oz (30 g) honey or maple syrup
- 1 tsp vanilla extract
- Pinch of salt
- 2 oz (60 g) dark chocolate (70% cocoa or higher)
- 1 tsp coconut oil

Directions:

1. In a bowl, combine the chia seeds and unsweetened shredded coconut.
2. In a small saucepan, warm the coconut milk over low heat. Stir in the honey or maple syrup, vanilla extract, and a pinch of salt until well combined.
3. Pour the coconut milk mixture over the chia seed-coconut mixture and mix until everything is well incorporated. Let the mixture sit for about 10 minutes to allow the chia seeds to absorb the liquid.
4. Preheat the oven to 325°F (160°C) and line a baking sheet with parchment paper.
5. Using your hands, form the chia-coconut mixture into small macaroon-sized rounds and place them on the prepared baking sheet.
6. Bake in the preheated oven for about 15-20 minutes or until the macaroons are golden brown on the edges.
7. In a microwave-safe bowl, melt the dark chocolate and coconut oil together in 20-second intervals, stirring until smooth.
8. Drizzle the melted chocolate over the cooled chia seed coconut macaroons.
9. Allow the chocolate to set before serving.

Nutritional Values: Calories: 180 kcal | Fat: 11 g | Protein: 3 g | Carbs: 18 g | Net carbs: 14 g | Fiber: 4 g | Cholesterol: 0 mg | Sodium: 15 mg | Potassium: 190 mg

Useful Tip: Make sure to let the chia seed and coconut mixture sit for about 10 minutes before shaping the macaroons. This allows the chia seeds to absorb the liquid and helps bind the mixture together. These Chia Seed Coconut Macaroons with Dark Chocolate Drizzle are a delightful and wholesome treat, providing a balance of healthy fats, fiber, and a touch of indulgence from the dark chocolate. Enjoy them as a satisfying snack or dessert option while following the GOLO Diet.

Roasted Cherry Vanilla Parfait with Almond Crumble

Serving: 4 | Prep time: 15 minutes | Cook time: 20 minutes

Ingredients:

- 12 oz (340 g) fresh cherries, pitted and halved
- 2 tsp honey or maple syrup
- 1 tsp vanilla extract
- 4 oz (115 g) almond flour
- 2 tbsp coconut oil, melted
- 1 tsp cinnamon
- 6 oz (450 g) Greek yogurt
- 1 tsp vanilla extract
- 2 oz (60 g) sliced almonds, toasted

Directions:

1. Preheat the oven to 375°F (190°C).
2. In a bowl, toss the fresh cherry halves with honey (or maple syrup) and vanilla extract until well coated. Spread them on a baking sheet in a single layer and roast for about 15-20 minutes or until the cherries are softened and slightly caramelized. Allow them to cool.
3. In another bowl, combine almond flour, melted coconut oil, and cinnamon to create the almond crumble mixture.
4. Spread the almond crumble mixture on a parchment-lined baking sheet and bake for about 8-10 minutes or until golden brown and crispy. Let it cool and break it into smaller crumbles.
5. In a separate bowl, mix Greek yogurt and vanilla extract until smooth and creamy.
6. To assemble the parfaits, layer roasted cherry halves, Greek yogurt mixture, and almond crumble in serving glasses or bowls.
7. Top each parfait with a sprinkle of toasted sliced almonds.
8. Serve immediately or refrigerate until ready to enjoy.

Nutritional Values: Calories: 250 kcal | Fat: 15 g | Protein: 10 g | Carbs: 20 g | Net carbs: 12 g | Fiber: 8 g | Cholesterol: 10 mg | Sodium: 40 mg | Potassium: 340 mg

Useful Tip: To enhance the flavor of the almond crumble, consider adding a pinch of sea salt or a drizzle of honey before baking. This Roasted Cherry Vanilla Parfait with Almond Crumble is a satisfying and nutrient-rich dessert option that combines the natural sweetness of roasted cherries with the crunch of almond crumble and the creaminess of Greek yogurt, making it a delightful treat while adhering to the GOLO Diet principles. Enjoy the harmony of flavors and textures in this balanced dessert!

Pistachio Date Truffles with Cardamom and Rose Water

Serving: 4 | Prep time: 20 minutes | Cook time: 0 minutes

Ingredients:

- 5 oz (140 g) pitted dates
- 2 oz (60 g) shelled pistachios
- 1/2 tsp ground cardamom
- 1/2 tsp rose water
- 1 oz (30 g) unsweetened shredded coconut
- 1 oz (30 g) dark chocolate, melted
- 1 tsp coconut oil

Directions:

1. In a food processor, combine pitted dates, shelled pistachios, ground cardamom, and rose water. Pulse until the mixture comes together and forms a sticky dough.
2. Scoop out small portions of the mixture and roll them into bite-sized truffles using your hands.
3. Spread the unsweetened shredded coconut on a plate. Roll each truffle in the coconut to coat evenly.
4. In a microwave-safe bowl, melt the dark chocolate and coconut oil together in 20-second intervals, stirring until smooth.
5. Using a fork, drizzle the melted chocolate over the coconut-coated truffles.
6. Place the truffles on a parchment-lined tray and refrigerate for about 15-20 minutes to allow the chocolate to set.
7. Once the chocolate is set, transfer the truffles to an airtight container and store them in the refrigerator until ready to serve.

Nutritional Values: Calories: 120 kcal | Fat: 6 g | Protein: 2 g | Carbs: 16 g | Net carbs: 13 g | Fiber: 3 g | Cholesterol: 0 mg | Sodium: 5 mg | Potassium: 200 mg

Useful Tip: For an extra layer of flavor, you can roll the truffles in a mixture of crushed pistachios and a touch of ground cardamom before coating them with shredded coconut. These Pistachio Date Truffles with Cardamom and Rose Water are a delightful and nutritious treat that combines the sweetness of dates with the earthiness of pistachios, elevated by the aromatic notes of cardamom and rose water, making them a perfect snack or dessert option that aligns with the GOLO Diet principles. Enjoy the exotic flavors and satisfying texture of these truffles guilt-free!

Tropical Mango Sorbet with Lime Zest and Mint Leaves

Serving: 4 | Prep time: 15 minutes | Cook time: 0 minutes

Ingredients:

- 16 oz (450 g) frozen mango chunks
- 2 oz (60 ml) lime juice
- Zest of 1 lime
- 2 oz (60 ml) coconut water
- 2 tbsp honey or agave syrup (adjust to taste)
- Fresh mint leaves, for garnish

Directions:

1. In a high-speed blender or food processor, combine the frozen mango chunks, lime juice, lime zest, coconut water, and honey or agave syrup.
2. Blend the mixture until smooth and creamy, scraping down the sides as needed.
3. Taste and adjust the sweetness if desired by adding more honey or agave syrup.
4. Transfer the sorbet mixture to a shallow, freezer-safe container and spread it evenly.
5. Cover the container with plastic wrap or a lid and place it in the freezer for at least 3-4 hours or until the sorbet is firm.
6. Once the sorbet is firm, scoop it into serving bowls and garnish with fresh mint leaves.
7. Allow the sorbet to sit at room temperature for a few minutes before serving to soften slightly.
8. Enjoy the refreshing and tropical flavors of the Mango Sorbet with the zesty kick of lime and the aromatic touch of mint leaves.

Nutritional Values: Calories: 120 kcal | Fat: 0.5 g | Protein: 1 g | Carbs: 30 g | Net carbs: 26 g | Fiber: 4 g | Cholesterol: 0 mg | Sodium: 10 mg | Potassium: 280 mg

Useful Tip: To enhance the tropical experience, consider adding a sprinkle of toasted coconut flakes on top of the sorbet before serving. The combination of sweet mango, tangy lime, and refreshing mint makes this Tropical Mango Sorbet with Lime Zest and Mint Leaves a delightful and guilt-free dessert option that aligns with the GOLO Diet principles. Enjoy the natural sweetness and vibrant flavors of this treat while staying on track with your healthy eating goals.

Chocolate Peanut Butter Chia Pudding with Crushed Pretzels

Serving: 4 | Prep Time: 15 minutes | Cook Time: 0 minutes

Ingredients:

- 2 oz (56 g) chia seeds
- 2 oz (56 g) unsweetened cocoa powder
- 4 oz (113 g) natural peanut butter
- 12 oz (355 ml) unsweetened almond milk
- 2 oz (56 g) crushed pretzels
- 1 oz (28 g) dark chocolate chips
- 1 tbsp honey (optional, for added sweetness)
- 1 tsp vanilla extract

Directions:

1. In a mixing bowl, combine chia seeds and cocoa powder.
2. Stir in the natural peanut butter until well incorporated.
3. Gradually pour in the unsweetened almond milk while stirring to avoid clumps.
4. Add honey (if using) and vanilla extract, and mix until the mixture is smooth and consistent.
5. Allow the mixture to sit for about 10 minutes, giving the chia seeds time to absorb the liquid and thicken the pudding.
6. Once the pudding has thickened, give it a good stir to ensure an even texture.
7. Divide the pudding into serving glasses or bowls.
8. In a resealable plastic bag, crush the pretzels into small pieces.
9. Sprinkle the crushed pretzels over the top of each pudding serving.
10. Finish by adding a sprinkle of dark chocolate chips for an extra touch of indulgence.
11. Refrigerate the puddings for at least 1 hour before serving to allow the flavors to meld.
12. Enjoy the rich and creamy Chocolate Peanut Butter Chia Pudding with a delightful crunch from the crushed pretzels.

Nutritional Values: Calories: 290 kcal | Fat: 18 g | Protein: 10 g | Carbs: 25 g | Net Carbs: 13 g | Fiber: 12 g | Cholesterol: 0 mg | Sodium: 255 mg | Potassium: 325 mg

Useful Tip: For a variation, you can add sliced bananas or fresh berries on top of the pudding for a fruity twist.

Baked Cinnamon Sugar Plantains with Greek Yogurt Dip

Serving: 4 | Prep Time: 10 minutes | Cook Time: 20 minutes

Ingredients:

- 16 oz (453 g) ripe plantains (about 2 plantains), peeled and sliced diagonally
- 2 tbsp coconut oil, melted
- 1 tbsp granulated sugar substitute (e.g., erythritol)
- 1 tsp ground cinnamon
- Pinch of salt
- 8 oz (227 g) Greek yogurt
- 1 tsp honey (optional, for the dip)
- 1/2 tsp vanilla extract

Directions:

1. Preheat the oven to 375°F (190°C) and line a baking sheet with parchment paper.
2. In a large bowl, toss the sliced plantains with melted coconut oil until well coated.
3. In a separate small bowl, mix the granulated sugar substitute, ground cinnamon, and a pinch of salt.
4. Sprinkle the cinnamon sugar mixture over the plantain slices and gently toss to evenly coat.
5. Arrange the coated plantains on the prepared baking sheet in a single layer.
6. Bake in the preheated oven for about 20 minutes, flipping the slices halfway through, until the plantains are golden and slightly crispy.
7. While the plantains are baking, prepare the Greek yogurt dip. In a bowl, mix the Greek yogurt, honey (if using), and vanilla extract until smooth.
8. Once the plantains are done baking, remove them from the oven and let them cool slightly.
9. Serve the baked cinnamon sugar plantains alongside the Greek yogurt dip.
10. Dip the warm plantain slices into the cool and creamy Greek yogurt dip, and enjoy the delightful contrast of flavors and textures.

Nutritional Values: Calories: 190 kcal | Fat: 7 g | Protein: 6 g | Carbs: 30 g | Net Carbs: 21 g | Fiber: 9 g | Cholesterol: 5 mg | Sodium: 40 mg | Potassium: 510 mg

Useful Tip: For an extra crunch, you can sprinkle some crushed nuts, such as almonds or walnuts, over the baked plantains before serving.

Blueberry Almond Biscotti with Lemon Zest

Serving: 4 | Prep Time: 15 minutes | Cook Time: 30 minutes

Ingredients:

- 6 oz (170 g) almond flour
- 2 oz (56 g) dried blueberries
- 1 oz (28 g) chopped almonds
- 1 oz (28 g) granulated sugar substitute (e.g., monk fruit sweetener)
- Zest of 1 lemon
- 2 large eggs
- 1 tsp vanilla extract
- Pinch of salt
- 1 tsp baking powder

Directions:

1. Preheat the oven to 325°F (165°C) and line a baking sheet with parchment paper.
2. In a large mixing bowl, combine almond flour, dried blueberries, chopped almonds, granulated sugar substitute, baking powder, and the zest of 1 lemon.
3. In a separate bowl, whisk together the eggs, vanilla extract, and a pinch of salt until well blended.
4. Gradually add the wet ingredients to the dry ingredients and mix until a dough forms.
5. Divide the dough in half and shape each portion into a log, about 8 inches long and 1 inch wide.
6. Place the logs on the prepared baking sheet, leaving space between them.
7. Bake in the preheated oven for 20-25 minutes, or until the logs are firm to the touch and lightly golden.
8. Remove the logs from the oven and let them cool on the baking sheet for about 10 minutes.
9. Reduce the oven temperature to 300°F (150°C).
10. Once the logs are slightly cooled, carefully transfer them to a cutting board and use a sharp knife to cut them into diagonal slices, about 1/2 inch wide.
11. Place the slices back on the baking sheet and bake for an additional 10-15 minutes, turning them halfway through, until they are crisp and golden.
12. Allow the biscotti to cool completely before serving.

Nutritional Values: Calories: 180 kcal | Fat: 15 g | Protein: 6 g | Carbs: 7 g | Net Carbs: 3 g | Fiber: 4 g | Cholesterol: 80 mg | Sodium: 50 mg | Potassium: 160 mg

Useful Tip: For a tangy twist, drizzle melted dark chocolate over the cooled biscotti before serving.

Tropical Turmeric Smoothie with Pineapple and Mango

Serving: 4 | Prep Time: 10 minutes | Cook Time: 0 minutes

Ingredients:

- 10 oz (283 g) frozen pineapple chunks
- 10 oz (283 g) frozen mango chunks
- 1 large banana, peeled and sliced
- 1 tsp ground turmeric
- 1/2 tsp ground ginger
- 16 oz (473 ml) unsweetened coconut milk
- 2 tbsp lime juice
- 1 tbsp honey (optional, for added sweetness)
- 1/2 tsp vanilla extract

Directions:

1. In a blender, combine the frozen pineapple chunks, frozen mango chunks, sliced banana, ground turmeric, ground ginger, unsweetened coconut milk, lime juice, honey (if using), and vanilla extract.
2. Blend on high until all the ingredients are well combined and the smoothie is creamy and smooth.
3. Taste and adjust sweetness by adding more honey, if desired.
4. If the smoothie is too thick, you can add a bit more coconut milk to achieve your preferred consistency.
5. Pour the tropical turmeric smoothie into glasses and garnish with a slice of lime or a sprinkle of ground turmeric, if desired.
6. Serve immediately and savor the refreshing and vibrant flavors of this tropical treat.

Nutritional Values: Calories: 150 kcal | Fat: 6 g | Protein: 1 g | Carbs: 27 g | Net Carbs: 20 g | Fiber: 7 g | Cholesterol: 0 mg | Sodium: 35 mg | Potassium: 300 mg

Useful Tip: For an extra boost of nutrition, consider adding a scoop of your favorite plant-based protein powder to the smoothie.

Blueberry Basil Infused Water with Lemon and Mint

Serving: 4 | Prep Time: 5 minutes | Cook Time: 0 minutes

Ingredients:

- 5.3 oz (150 g) fresh blueberries
- 1 small lemon, thinly sliced
- 1 small bunch fresh basil leaves
- 1 small bunch fresh mint leaves
- 32 oz (946 ml) filtered water
- Ice cubes, for serving

Directions:

1. In a pitcher, combine the fresh blueberries, thinly sliced lemon, fresh basil leaves, and fresh mint leaves.
2. Gently muddle the ingredients with a muddler or the back of a spoon to release their flavors.
3. Fill the pitcher with 32 oz (946 ml) of filtered water.
4. Stir the mixture gently to distribute the flavors throughout the water.
5. Cover the pitcher and refrigerate for at least 2 hours, or ideally overnight, to allow the flavors to infuse.
6. When serving, you can either strain the infused water into glasses or pour it directly, allowing the fruits and herbs to float in the water.
7. Add ice cubes to each glass if desired.
8. Enjoy the refreshing and hydrating Blueberry Basil Infused Water with a touch of lemon and mint.

Nutritional Values: Calories: 10 kcal | Fat: 0 g | Protein: 0 g | Carbs: 3 g | Net Carbs: 2 g | Fiber: 1 g | Cholesterol: 0 mg | Sodium: 5 mg | Potassium: 45 mg

Useful Tip: Reuse the infused fruits and herbs for a second batch of water to maximize the flavors and reduce waste.

Green Apple and Ginger Detox Juice with Cucumber

Serving: 4 | Prep Time: 10 minutes | Cook Time: 0 minutes

Ingredients:

- 2 medium green apples, cored and cut into chunks
- 1 cucumber, peeled and cut into chunks
- 1 oz (28 g) fresh ginger, peeled and chopped
- 1 lemon, peeled and segmented
- 32 oz (946 ml) filtered water
- Ice cubes, for serving

Directions:

1. In a juicer, process the green apple chunks, cucumber chunks, fresh ginger, and lemon segments.
2. Collect the freshly extracted juice in a pitcher.
3. Stir in 32 oz (946 ml) of filtered water to dilute the juice and create a refreshing and hydrating detox beverage.
4. Mix well to ensure the flavors are evenly distributed.
5. Fill glasses with ice cubes and pour the Green Apple and Ginger Detox Juice over the ice.
6. Give the juice a quick stir before enjoying the invigorating flavors.

Nutritional Values: Calories: 70 kcal | Fat: 0 g | Protein: 1 g | Carbs: 18 g | Net Carbs: 14 g | Fiber: 4 g | Cholesterol: 0 mg | Sodium: 5 mg | Potassium: 330 mg

Useful Tip: For an extra boost of antioxidants, consider adding a handful of fresh spinach or kale to the juicer for added nutrient content.

Hibiscus Berry Iced Tea with Fresh Berries and Lemon

Serving: 4 | Prep Time: 5 minutes | Cook Time: 10 minutes (plus cooling time)

Ingredients:

- 0.7 oz (20 g) dried hibiscus flowers
- 32 oz (946 ml) filtered water
- 1 oz (28 g) mixed fresh berries (such as strawberries, blueberries, raspberries)
- 1 lemon, thinly sliced
- 1 tbsp honey (optional, for added sweetness)
- Fresh mint leaves, for garnish
- Ice cubes, for serving

Directions:

1. In a medium saucepan, bring 32 oz (946 ml) of filtered water to a boil.
2. Remove the saucepan from heat and add the dried hibiscus flowers.
3. Allow the hibiscus flowers to steep in the hot water for about 10 minutes.
4. After steeping, strain the hibiscus tea into a pitcher and let it cool to room temperature.
5. Once the tea has cooled, refrigerate it until chilled.
6. To serve, fill glasses with ice cubes and pour the chilled hibiscus tea over the ice.
7. Add a handful of mixed fresh berries and a few lemon slices to each glass.
8. If desired, drizzle honey into each glass for added sweetness.
9. Garnish with fresh mint leaves for a burst of aromatic freshness.
10. Stir the tea gently to combine the flavors, and enjoy the vibrant and refreshing Hibiscus Berry Iced Tea.

Nutritional Values: Calories: 20 kcal | Fat: 0 g | Protein: 0 g | Carbs: 5 g | Net Carbs: 4 g | Fiber: 1 g | Cholesterol: 0 mg | Sodium: 5 mg | Potassium: 30 mg

Useful Tip: For an even more intense berry flavor, consider muddling a few berries at the bottom of each glass before adding the ice and hibiscus tea.

Creamy Matcha Latte with Almond Milk and Honey

Serving: 1 | Prep Time: 5 minutes | Cook Time: 5 minutes

Ingredients:

- 1 tsp matcha green tea powder
- 4 oz (120 ml) unsweetened almond milk
- 4 oz (120 ml) hot water (not boiling)
- 1 tsp honey (or sweetener of choice)
- Optional: a pinch of cinnamon or nutmeg for garnish

Directions:

1. In a small bowl, sift the matcha green tea powder to remove any lumps.
2. In a separate cup, heat the almond milk until warm (not boiling).
3. In another cup, heat the water until it's hot but not boiling.
4. In a mug, combine the sifted matcha powder and the hot water.
5. Use a whisk or a matcha whisk to vigorously whisk the matcha and water until it's well combined and frothy.
6. Pour the warmed almond milk into the mug with the matcha mixture.
7. Add honey (or sweetener of choice) and stir until the honey is dissolved and the mixture is creamy.
8. If desired, sprinkle a pinch of cinnamon or nutmeg on top for extra flavor.
9. Enjoy your Creamy Matcha Latte, savoring the earthy and vibrant notes of matcha with a touch of sweetness.

Nutritional Values: Calories: 30 kcal | Fat: 1 g | Protein: 1 g | Carbs: 4 g | Net Carbs: 3 g | Fiber: 1 g | Cholesterol: 0 mg | Sodium: 150 mg | Potassium: 60 mg

Useful Tip: For an iced version, let the matcha mixture cool after whisking, then pour it over ice and cold almond milk.

Sparkling Raspberry Limeade with Fresh Mint Leaves

Serving: 4 | Prep Time: 10 minutes | Cook Time: 0 minutes

Ingredients:

- 5.3 oz (150 g) fresh raspberries
- 2 limes, juiced
- 0.7 oz (20 g) fresh mint leaves
- 32 oz (946 ml) sparkling water
- 1-2 tbsp honey (adjust to taste)
- Ice cubes, for serving

Directions:

1. In a pitcher, muddle the fresh raspberries to release their juices and flavor.
2. Add the freshly squeezed lime juice to the pitcher.
3. Gently crush the fresh mint leaves in your hands to release their aroma, then add them to the pitcher.
4. Pour the sparkling water into the pitcher, and gently stir to combine the ingredients.
5. Add honey to the mixture and stir until it's dissolved and well mixed (adjust sweetness to taste).
6. Fill glasses with ice cubes and pour the Sparkling Raspberry Limeade over the ice.
7. Garnish each glass with a sprig of fresh mint and a few extra raspberries, if desired.
8. Stir gently to distribute the flavors, and enjoy the refreshing and effervescent Raspberry Limeade.

Nutritional Values: Calories: 30 kcal | Fat: 0 g | Protein: 0 g | Carbs: 8 g | Net Carbs: 7 g | Fiber: 1 g | Cholesterol: 0 mg | Sodium: 0 mg | Potassium: 50 mg

Useful Tip: For a fancier presentation, freeze raspberries and lime slices in ice cube trays to make fruit-infused ice cubes that won't dilute your drink.

Chai Spiced Golden Milk Latte with Turmeric and Cinnamon

Serving: 1 | Prep Time: 5 minutes | Cook Time: 5 minutes

Ingredients:

- 1 tsp ground turmeric
- 1/2 tsp ground cinnamon
- 1/4 tsp ground ginger
- 1/4 tsp ground cardamom
- Pinch of black pepper
- 8 oz (240 ml) unsweetened almond milk
- 4 oz (120 ml) hot water
- 1 tsp honey (optional, for added sweetness)
- 1/2 tsp vanilla extract

Directions:

1. In a small bowl, mix together the ground turmeric, ground cinnamon, ground ginger, ground cardamom, and a pinch of black pepper.
2. In a small saucepan, heat the almond milk until warm (not boiling).
3. In another cup, heat the water until it's hot but not boiling.
4. In a mug, combine 1 teaspoon of the chai spice mixture with the hot water.
5. Use a whisk to blend the chai spice mixture and hot water until smooth.
6. Pour the warmed almond milk into the mug with the chai mixture.
7. Add honey (if using) and vanilla extract, and stir until the honey is dissolved and the mixture is well combined.
8. Enjoy your Chai Spiced Golden Milk Latte, relishing the warm and comforting blend of spices and the goodness of turmeric.

Nutritional Values: Calories: 40 kcal | Fat: 1.5 g | Protein: 1 g | Carbs: 7 g | Net Carbs: 6 g | Fiber: 1 g | Cholesterol: 0 mg | Sodium: 160 mg | Potassium: 80 mg

Useful Tip: If you prefer a creamier latte, you can use coconut milk instead of almond milk for a richer texture and flavor.

Cucumber and Lime Electrolyte Refresher with Sea Salt

Serving: 1 | Prep Time: 5 minutes | Cook Time: 0 minutes

Ingredients:

- 5.3 oz (150 g) cucumber, peeled and sliced
- 1 lime, juiced
- 16 oz (473 ml) filtered water
- Pinch of high-quality sea salt
- Ice cubes, for serving

Directions:

1. In a blender, combine the cucumber slices and freshly squeezed lime juice.
2. Blend until the cucumber is completely pureed.
3. Strain the cucumber-lime mixture through a fine mesh strainer into a glass or pitcher.
4. Add 16 oz (473 ml) of filtered water to the strained mixture.
5. Add a pinch of high-quality sea salt to the mixture and stir well to dissolve.
6. Fill a glass with ice cubes and pour the Cucumber and Lime Electrolyte Refresher over the ice.
7. Stir gently to distribute the flavors and salt.
8. Sip and savor the refreshing and hydrating blend that helps replenish electrolytes.

Nutritional Values: Calories: 10 kcal | Fat: 0 g | Protein: 0 g | Carbs: 3 g | Net Carbs: 2 g | Fiber: 1 g | Cholesterol: 0 mg | Sodium: 300 mg | Potassium: 200 mg

Useful Tip: For an extra boost of natural sweetness and electrolytes, consider adding a splash of coconut water to the refresher.

Watermelon Rosemary Lemonade with a Hint of Agave

Serving: 4 | Prep Time: 10 minutes | Cook Time: 0 minutes

Ingredients:

- 20 oz (567 g) fresh watermelon, cubed
- 2 sprigs fresh rosemary
- 2 lemons, juiced
- 1-2 tbsp agave nectar (adjust to taste)
- 32 oz (946 ml) filtered water
- Ice cubes, for serving
- Additional rosemary sprigs and lemon slices for garnish

Directions:

1. In a blender, puree the fresh watermelon cubes until smooth.
2. Strain the watermelon puree through a fine mesh strainer into a pitcher to remove any pulp.
3. Gently muddle one sprig of fresh rosemary to release its aroma, then add it to the pitcher.
4. Add the freshly squeezed lemon juice to the pitcher.
5. Stir in the agave nectar, adjusting the amount to achieve your desired level of sweetness.
6. Add 32 oz (946 ml) of filtered water to the mixture and stir well.
7. Fill glasses with ice cubes and pour the Watermelon Rosemary Lemonade over the ice.
8. Garnish each glass with a sprig of rosemary and a slice of lemon.
9. Give the lemonade a gentle stir before enjoying the refreshing blend of watermelon, rosemary, and citrus.

Nutritional Values: Calories: 50 kcal | Fat: 0 g | Protein: 1 g | Carbs: 13 g | Net Carbs: 12 g | Fiber: 1 g | Cholesterol: 0 mg | Sodium: 5 mg | Potassium: 200 mg

Useful Tip: For a unique twist, consider adding a splash of sparkling water to each glass for a fizzy version of this delightful lemonade.

Начало формы

Coconut Mango Lassi Smoothie with Cardamom and Almonds

Serving: 2 | Prep Time: 10 minutes | Cook Time: 0 minutes

Ingredients:

- 7 oz (200 g) ripe mango, peeled and diced
- 4 oz (120 ml) unsweetened coconut milk
- 4 oz (120 ml) plain Greek yogurt
- 1/4 tsp ground cardamom
- 1 tbsp almonds, chopped
- 1 tsp honey (optional, for added sweetness)
- Ice cubes, for serving

Directions:

1. In a blender, combine the diced mango, unsweetened coconut milk, plain Greek yogurt, and ground cardamom.
2. Blend until the mixture is smooth and creamy.
3. Taste the smoothie and add honey if desired for a touch of sweetness (adjust to taste).
4. Add a handful of ice cubes to the blender and blend again until the smoothie is chilled and frothy.
5. Pour the Coconut Mango Lassi Smoothie into glasses.
6. Garnish each glass with chopped almonds for added crunch and a sprinkle of ground cardamom for extra flavor.
7. Sip and enjoy the tropical flavors of the Coconut Mango Lassi Smoothie with a delightful hint of cardamom.

Nutritional Values: Calories: 150 kcal | Fat: 7 g | Protein: 7 g | Carbs: 18 g | Net Carbs: 15 g | Fiber: 3 g | Cholesterol: 5 mg | Sodium: 30 mg | Potassium: 280 mg

Useful Tip: For a dairy-free version, you can use dairy-free yogurt or coconut yogurt instead of Greek yogurt.

Meal Plan

Week 1: Meal Plan

Day 1:
- **Breakfast:** Almond Butter Banana Pancakes
- **Lunch:** Mediterranean Chickpea Salad with Lemon Herb Dressing
- **Snacks:** Cucumber and Hummus Stuffed Mini Bell Peppers / Crunchy Kale Chips with Nutritional Yeast
- **Dinner:** Lemon Thyme Grilled Turkey Cutlets with Zucchini Noodles

Day 2:
- **Breakfast:** Chia Berry Breakfast Parfait
- **Lunch:** Roasted Sweet Potato and Kale Salad with Tahini Drizzle
- **Snacks:** Zucchini Fritters with Lemon-Herb Greek Yogurt Dip / Coconut-Covered Date and Nut Energy Balls
- **Dinner:** Sesame Ginger Glazed Chicken Skewers with Cauliflower Rice

Day 3:
- **Breakfast:** Sweet Potato Hash with Turkey Sausage
- **Lunch:** Thai-Inspired Quinoa Salad with Peanut Lime Dressing
- **Snacks:** Baked Sweet Potato Fries with Cumin and Paprika / Mashed Avocado and Tomato Bruschetta on Whole Wheat Crackers
- **Dinner:** Spiced Paprika Chicken Thighs with Roasted Brussels Sprouts

Day 4:
- **Breakfast:** Cinnamon Raisin Oatmeal with Pecans
- **Lunch:** Creamy Broccoli and Cauliflower Soup with Garlic Parmesan Croutons
- **Snacks:** Spicy Edamame and Sesame Snack Mix / Roasted Butternut Squash and Black Bean Taco Filling (used as a dip)
- **Dinner:** Orange Rosemary Baked Quail with Sautéed Spinach

Day 5:
- **Breakfast:** Spinach and Feta Egg White Scramble
- **Lunch:** Roasted Cauliflower and Chickpea Salad with Turmeric Tahini
- **Snacks:** Smoked Salmon Cucumber Bites with Dill Cream Cheese / Lentil and Vegetable Stir-Fry with Quinoa (used as a dip)
- **Dinner:** Crispy Dijon Mustard Chicken Tenders with Roasted Asparagus

Day 6:
- **Breakfast:** Blueberry Coconut Flour Waffles
- **Lunch:** Mexican Street Corn Salad with Chili Lime Dressing
- **Snacks:** Spaghetti Squash Pad Thai with Peanut Sauce and Tofu (rolled in lettuce leaves) / Spicy Tuna Lettuce Wraps with Avocado and Sriracha Mayo
- **Dinner:** Coconut Curry Chicken Stir-Fry with Cauliflower Rice

Day 7:
- **Breakfast:** Zucchini and Mushroom Breakfast Quesadilla
- **Lunch:** Grilled Chicken Caesar Salad with Creamy Avocado Dressing
- **Snacks:** Vegan Black Bean Chili with Cornbread Muffins (used as a topping) / Vegan Mediterranean Pizza with Cauliflower Crust and Hummus Spread (cut into smaller pieces)
- **Dinner:** Honey Sriracha Glazed Turkey Meatballs with Steamed Broccoli

Week 2: Meal Plan

Day 8:
- **Breakfast:** Apple Cinnamon Breakfast Quinoa
- **Lunch:** Tuna Nicoise Salad with Lemon Herb Vinaigrette
- **Snacks:** Zucchini Noodles with Creamy Avocado Pesto and Cherry Tomatoes (used as a cold salad) / Cucumber and Hummus Stuffed Mini Bell Peppers
- **Dinner:** Mango Chipotle Grilled Chicken Breast with Cilantro Lime Cauliflower Rice

Day 9:
- **Breakfast:** Mediterranean-style Veggie Omelette
- **Lunch:** Roasted Butternut Squash and Pomegranate Salad with Maple Dijon Dressing
- **Snacks:** Mediterranean Stuffed Bell Peppers with Quinoa and Olives (used as a snack-sized version) / Crunchy Kale Chips with Nutritional Yeast
- **Dinner:** Garlic Parmesan Crusted Chicken with Roasted Carrots

Day 10:
- **Breakfast:** Bacon and Spinach Stuffed Portobello Mushrooms
- **Lunch:** Roasted Brussels Sprouts and Quinoa Salad with Lemon Mustard Dressing
- **Snacks:** Roasted Beet and Orange Salad with Arugula and Maple-Mustard Dressing (used as a cold salad) / Coconut-Covered Date and Nut Energy Balls
- **Dinner:** Tender Herb-Marinated Pork Chops with Lemon Herb Green Beans

Day 11:
- **Breakfast:** Flaxseed Banana Muffins with Walnuts
- **Lunch:** Thai Coconut Chicken Soup with Lemongrass and Lime
- **Snacks:** Spicy Chickpea and Spinach Curry with Fragrant Basmati Rice (used as a filling for lettuce wraps) / Mashed Avocado and Tomato Bruschetta on Whole Wheat Crackers
- **Dinner:** Spiced Lamb Meatballs with Cumin-Scented Cauliflower Rice

Day 12:
- **Breakfast:** Smoked Salmon and Cream Cheese Stuffed Bell Peppers
- **Lunch:** Herb-Crusted Baked Lobster Tail with Garlic Mashed Cauliflower
- **Snacks:** Cauliflower Rice Stir-Fry with Tofu and Ginger-Sesame Sauce (used as a cold salad) / Baked Sweet Potato Fries with Cumin and Paprika
- **Dinner:** Savory Rosemary Roast Beef with Sautéed Mushrooms and Asparagus

Day 13:
- **Breakfast:** Turmeric Infused Golden Omelette
- **Lunch:** Lemon Dill Garlic Butter Crab Cakes with Asparagus Spears
- **Snacks:** Vegan Spinach and Artichoke Stuffed Portobello Mushrooms (cut into smaller pieces) / Roasted Butternut Squash and Black Bean Taco Filling (used as a topping)
- **Dinner:** Chimichurri Marinated Grilled Pork Tenderloin with Roasted Brussels Sprouts

Day 14:
- **Breakfast:** Quinoa and Black Bean Breakfast Burrito
- **Lunch:** Herb-Marinated Grilled Trout with Lemon-Dill Sauce
- **Snacks:** Grilled Eggplant and Zucchini Roll-Ups with Sun-Dried Tomato Pesto / Smoked Salmon Cucumber Bites with Dill Cream Cheese
- **Dinner:** Tender Ginger-Soy Marinated Beef Stir-Fry with Cauliflower Rice

Day 15:
- **Breakfast:** Mango Coconut Breakfast Rice Bowl
- **Lunch:** Lentil and Vegetable Stir-Fry with Quinoa and Ginger-Sesame Sauce
- **Snacks:** Mediterranean Chickpea and Quinoa Bowl with Lemon-Herb Vinaigrette (used as a cold salad) / Zucchini Fritters with Lemon-Herb Greek Yogurt Dip
- **Dinner:** Balsamic Glazed Lamb Meatballs with Mediterranean Roasted Eggplant

Day 16:
- **Breakfast:** Broccoli and Cheese Egg Muffins
- **Lunch:** Moroccan Chickpea and Vegetable Tagine with Apricots and Almonds
- **Snacks:** Baked Mini Meatballs with Roasted Cherry Tomatoes (used as a topping) / Cucumber and Hummus Stuffed Mini Bell Peppers
- **Dinner:** Spiced Paprika Pork Skewers with Zucchini and Red Pepper Medley

Day 17:
- **Breakfast:** Blueberry Lemon Poppy Seed Muffins
- **Lunch:** Vegan Mediterranean Pizza with Cauliflower Crust and Hummus Spread
- **Snacks:** Sweet Potato and Chickpea Curry with Coconut Milk and Curry Leaves (used as a dip) / Crunchy Kale Chips with Nutritional Yeast
- **Dinner:** Cumin-Spiced Grilled Beef Steak with Turmeric Cauliflower Mash

Day 18:
- **Breakfast:** Greek Yogurt Berry Parfait with Granola
- **Lunch:** Vegan Spinach and Artichoke Stuffed Portobello Mushrooms
- **Snacks:** Roasted Brussels Sprouts and Quinoa Salad with Balsamic Glaze (used as a cold salad) / Coconut-Covered Date and Nut Energy Balls
- **Dinner:** Honey Mustard Glazed Pork Ribs with Garlic Mashed Cauliflower

Day 19:
- **Breakfast:** Caramelized Onion and Spinach Breakfast Casserole
- **Lunch:** Sweet Potato and Chickpea Curry with Coconut Milk and Curry Leaves
- **Snacks:** Turmeric Infused Golden Omelette (cut into bite-sized pieces) / Mashed Avocado and Tomato Bruschetta on Whole Wheat Crackers
- **Dinner:** Chipotle-Marinated Grilled Beef Sirloin with Smoky Paprika Sweet Potatoes

Day 20:
- **Breakfast:** Avocado and Bacon Breakfast Tacos
- **Lunch:** Grilled Eggplant and Zucchini Roll-Ups with Sun-Dried Tomato Pesto
- **Snacks:** Spicy Edamame and Sesame Snack Mix / Lentil and Vegetable Stir-Fry with Quinoa (used as a dip)
- **Dinner:** Herb-Crusted Baked Lobster Tail with Garlic Mashed Cauliflower

Day 21:
- **Breakfast:** Almond Butter Banana Pancakes
- **Lunch:** Mediterranean Chickpea and Quinoa Bowl with Lemon-Herb Vinaigrette
- **Snacks:** Vegan Lentil Shepherd's Pie with Mashed Sweet Potato Topping (used as a topping) / Smoked Salmon Cucumber Bites with Dill Cream Cheese
- **Dinner:** Thai Coconut Curry Mussels with Zucchini Noodles

Day 22:
- **Breakfast:** Chia Berry Breakfast Parfait
- **Lunch:** Roasted Beet and Goat Cheese Salad with Citrus Vinaigrette
- **Snacks:** Spaghetti Squash Pad Thai with Peanut Sauce and Tofu (used as a cold salad) / Zucchini Fritters with Lemon-Herb Greek Yogurt Dip
- **Dinner:** Lemon Thyme Grilled Turkey Cutlets with Zucchini Noodles

Day 23:
- **Breakfast:** Sweet Potato Hash with Turkey Sausage
- **Lunch:** Strawberry Spinach Salad with Poppy Seed Dressing
- **Snacks:** Vegan Black Bean Chili with Cornbread Muffins (used as a dip) / Cucumber and Hummus Stuffed Mini Bell Peppers
- **Dinner:** Spicy Grilled Tilapia with Mango Salsa

Day 24:
- **Breakfast:** Cinnamon Raisin Oatmeal with Pecans
- **Lunch:** Roasted Red Pepper and Tomato Soup with Basil Pesto Swirl
- **Snacks:** Moroccan Chickpea and Vegetable Tagine with Apricots and Almonds (used as a cold salad) / Coconut-Covered Date and Nut Energy Balls
- **Dinner:** Mediterranean-Style Grilled Sea Bass with Zucchini Noodles

Day 25:
- **Breakfast:** Spinach and Feta Egg White Scramble
- **Lunch:** Greek Cucumber and Feta Salad with Oregano Vinaigrette
- **Snacks:** Roasted Beet and Orange Salad with Arugula and Maple-Mustard Dressing (used as a cold salad) / Baked Sweet Potato Fries with Cumin and Paprika
- **Dinner:** Blackened Red Snapper Tacos with Avocado Crema

Day 26:
- **Breakfast:** Blueberry Coconut Flour Waffles
- **Lunch:** Apple Walnut Salad with Maple Dijon Dressing
- **Snacks:** Vegan Mediterranean Pizza with Cauliflower Crust and Hummus Spread (cut into smaller pieces) / Mashed Avocado and Tomato Bruschetta on Whole Wheat Crackers
- **Dinner:** Sesame Crusted Tuna Steaks with Cucumber Salad

Day 27:
- **Breakfast:** Zucchini and Mushroom Breakfast Quesadilla
- **Lunch:** Caprese Salad with Fresh Basil and Balsamic Glaze
- **Snacks:** Grilled Eggplant and Zucchini Roll-Ups with Sun-Dried Tomato Pesto / Lentil and Vegetable Stir-Fry with Quinoa (used as a dip)
- **Dinner:** Herb-Marinated Grilled Trout with Lemon-Dill Sauce

Day 28:
- **Breakfast:** Mango Coconut Breakfast Rice Bowl
- **Lunch:** Asian Sesame Chicken Salad with Ginger Soy Dressing
- **Snacks:** Cauliflower Rice Stir-Fry with Tofu and Ginger-Sesame Sauce (used as a cold salad) / Smoked Salmon Cucumber Bites with Dill Cream Cheese
- **Dinner:** Coconut Lime Grilled Halibut with Broccoli and Quinoa

Conclusion

As you close the pages of the Golo Diet Cookbook for Beginners, you've completed a transformative voyage into the world of balanced nutrition, mindful eating, and overall well-being. Throughout this culinary exploration, you've delved into the core principles of the Golo Diet, discovering the profound impact of insulin regulation, wholesome nutrition, and the Metabolic Fuel Matrix on your body and energy levels. The recipes within these pages have introduced you to diverse flavors and ingredients, empowering you to create meals that nourish your body and align with your wellness goals. From savory breakfasts to delectable desserts, each recipe embodies the essence of the Golo Diet's philosophy, demonstrating that healthy eating can be both satisfying and delicious. As you conclude this chapter of your journey, remember that the lessons and practices you've cultivated are not confined to these pages; they are a foundation upon which you can continue to build a lifestyle of vitality, energy, and well-being. The Golo Diet Cookbook has equipped you with culinary inspiration and paved the way for a future where mindful choices, balanced nutrition, and lasting wellness are your guiding stars.

As you turn the final pages of the Golo Diet Cookbook for Beginners, you're not just closing a book. Still, you're completing the first chapter of a transformative journey toward a healthier and more vibrant you. Throughout this cookbook, you've ventured into the world of the Golo Diet, uncovering its core principles and discovering the incredible impact that balanced nutrition and mindful eating can have on your overall well-being.

From the beginning, you've explored the concept of insulin regulation, understanding how it plays a pivotal role in maintaining stable blood sugar levels and preventing energy crashes and sugar cravings. The Golo Diet has shown you the power of choosing the right foods, managing carbohydrate intake, and creating a harmonious balance of nutrients to fuel your body optimally.

The journey didn't stop there. You dived into the heart of the Golo Diet, embracing the Metabolic Fuel Matrix that brought together proteins, fats, and carbohydrates in a symphony of nourishment. You've experienced the culinary delight of recipes meticulously crafted to maintain stable blood sugar levels, support your metabolism, and enhance your energy throughout the day.

Throughout the diverse array of recipes in this cookbook, you've witnessed the Golo Diet's commitment to wholesome nutrition. From hearty breakfasts to mouthwatering dinners and satisfying desserts, each recipe has been thoughtfully curated to ensure you enjoy flavors while prioritizing your well-being. This isn't just a cookbook; it's a guide to a balanced lifestyle that doesn't compromise on taste or health.

As you reflect on your journey, remember that the Golo Diet is more than just a temporary fix; it's a sustainable approach to health that encourages lifelong habits. It's not about deprivation or strict rules; it's about making mindful choices that empower you to take control of your wellness. The Golo Diet Cookbook for Beginners has provided you with the tools to continue creating nourishing, delicious meals that support your goals.

As you step away from these pages and back into your daily life, carry the knowledge you've gained. Whether you're enjoying a breakfast that stabilizes your energy, a lunch that keeps you satisfied, or a dinner that nourishes your body, the principles of the Golo Diet will remain your steadfast companion on your journey to a healthier you. You've set a foundation for lasting wellness, and the possibilities are endless as you explore the world of balanced nutrition, mindful eating, and vitality. Your journey with the Golo Diet Cookbook for Beginners is just the beginning of a vibrant chapter in your life, and the adventure awaits.

Made in the USA
Monee, IL
04 November 2023

45779828R00057